MAGNETIC RESONANCE IMAGING: BASIC PRINCIPLES

Second Edition

Magnetic Resonance Imaging: Basic Principles

Second Edition

Stuart W. Young, M.D.

Associate Professor of Diagnostic Radiology
Department of Diagnostic Radiology
Stanford University Medical Center
Stanford, California

Raven Press ☙ New York

Raven Press, 1185 Avenue of the Americas, New York, New York 10036

Made in the United States of America

The material contained in this volume was submitted as previously unpublished material, except in the instances in which credit has been given to the source from which some of the illustrative material was derived.

Great care has been taken to maintain the accuracy of the information contained in the volume. However, neither Raven Press nor the editors can be held responsible for errors or for any consequences arising from the use of the information contained herein.

Materials appearing in this book prepared by individuals as part of their official duties as U.S. Government employees are not covered by the above-mentioned copyright.

9 8 7 6 5 4 3 2 1

Library of Congress Cataloging-in-Publication Data

Young, Stuart W.
  Magnetic resonance imaging.

  Rev. ed. of: Nuclear magnetic resonance imaging.
© 1984.
  Bibliography: p. 244.
  Includes index.
  1. Magnetic resonance imaging.   I. Young, Stuart W.
Nuclear magnetic resonance imaging.   II. Title.
[DNLM: 1. Nuclear Magnetic Resonance—diagnostic use.
WN 445 Y76n]
RC78.7.N83Y68   1988   616.07'57   86-42889
ISBN 0-88167-366-8

To Susan

Preface

Rapid change is the common denominator in the field of magnetic resonance (MR). There are so many acronyms describing the various pulsing sequences that one can hardly keep track of them. There are now local coils designed for every part of the body. Developments in scanning hardware seem to change major portions of the magnetic resonance imaging (MRI) landscape overnight. Electrical shielding and resistive and permanent magnets have greatly simplified site preparation. Shielded gradients have markedly reduced eddy currents and improved image quality. New alloys offer the possibility of making superconducting magnets that will operate at room temperature or at the temperature of liquid nitrogen. The ability to image flow, chemical shift, and diffusion is now a reality. The field of *in vivo* localized magnetic resonance spectroscopy (MRS) ushered in by the large-bore MRI/MRS systems is experiencing explosive growth. Adding to the complexity are the new efforts toward containment of health-care costs, the entry of entrepreneurs into health-care delivery, the demographic changes among physician and patient populations, and the million-dollar-plus price tags for MRI scanners.

Basic principles in MRI are being redefined against this complex background. Effective practice of MRI requires the acquisition of new skills and understandings on an ongoing basis. In the second edition of this book I attempt to deal with some of these problems. The basic hardware and fundamentals of nuclear magnetic resonance (NMR) are discussed first. Conventional imaging sequences are then introduced before proceeding to the more complex sequences used to perform selective flow imaging and chemical-shift imaging. Because the MR signal is based on biochemical information, interpretation of the gray scale is complex and is dealt with in a separate chapter. The interdependence of the pulsing sequences and the tissue being evaluated are emphasized in this chapter. Head-to-foot clinical applications are presented to illustrate the value of MRI in clinical medicine, and a section illustrating MRI artifacts is included. An atlas of normal MRI anatomy follows the body of the text to provide additional anatomic detail as an aid in reviewing the images. In order to provide as broad an overview of MRI as possible, proton, chemical shift, ^{19}F, ^{23}Na, and ^{13}C images are included in this book and the images were obtained at 4.7, 2.1, 1.5, 0.38, and 0.3 Tesla using superconducting, resistive and permanent MRI scanners.

Chapters highlighting promising current research and the impact of the changing economic environment are placed together because many of the economic considerations and future technical developments in MRI are interdependent and mutually influential. These chapters deal more with the importance of macroeconomic factors in the practice of MRI than with an analysis of MRI operations and an emphasis on patient throughput.

Although there has been much progress, I believe that we are still on the threshold of this exciting technology. In X-ray and ultrasound imaging we were mainly anatomists detecting a disease after the anatomy had been altered by the disease. With MRI and localized *in vivo* MRS, the information contained in the MR signal is biochemical, and anatomic delineation is a fortunate consequence of the fact that clusters of biochemical similarities are defined by organs and tissues of similar types. We are just beginning to be able to manipulate and interpret the gray scale in MRI and understand the living biochemistry thereby revealed.

Stuart W. Young

Preface to the First Edition

This book has been organized to give an overview of the clinical and biological potential of nuclear magnetic resonance (NMR) imaging. It proceeds to discuss the fundamental principles of interaction of NMR and electromagnetic waves to generate the NMR signal on which NMR images are based. Subsequently, the components of the NMR signal, i.e., proton density, relaxation times (T_1 and T_2), and motion or flow, are introduced, together with their various interpretations and effects on image contrast.

Finally, some of the potential applications of NMR are introduced, as well as the types of imaging systems currently available. The book concludes with a chapter that considers the hazards of NMR imaging and site planning, and there is a bibliography for those desiring to do further reading in this area.

NMR imaging, in all likelihood, will become increasingly more important to a wide range of health professionals and investigators. This book has been compiled so that a broad spectrum of readers with general imaging or NMR background or biological and physiological medical backgrounds will be able to understand the basic principles of NMR imaging and progress to NMR studies in depth in their respective medical subspecialties. Health professionals who have been concerned with imaging subspecialties will benefit from becoming familiar with the physical principles of NMR, and those who have a background in NMR will further gain from the sections that are devoted to imaging and anatomic correlation. Finally, other health professionals without background in imaging or NMR should find the principles, as illustrated by analogies from common experience, helpful in understanding this complex technology.

Stuart W. Young

Acknowledgments

I am indebted to the faculty, fellows, residents, and graduate students of the many MRI and MRS programs at Stanford University who have contributed in many subtle and important ways to the quality of the images presented in this book. I should specifically like to mention Adam Ratner, M.D., Jeremy Rubin, M.D., Paul Chang, M.D., Dwight Nishimura, Ph.D., Bob DeLaPaz, M.D., Albert Macovski, Ph.D., Fred Burbank, M.D., David Sidenwurm, M.D., and Clark Carrol, M.D., of the Departments of Diagnostic Radiology and Electrical Engineering for their contributions.

William Bradley, M.D., Ph.D., Gary Fullerton, Ph.D., W. H. Oldendorf, M.D., Ph.D., Leon Partain, M.D., Ph.D., and Felix Wehrli, Ph.D., have provided invaluable assistance through their many publications and long hours of discussion in helping to develop the analogies used in this text.

For their generosity in allowing me to publish their research and MR images I am very grateful to the following: Paul A. Bottomley, Ph.D., Ralph E. Hurd, Ph.D., Linda K. Hutten, and The General Electric Company; Michael E. Moseley, Ph.D., Department of Radiology, University of California, San Francisco; Steven Quay, M.D., Ph.D., Salutar, Inc.; Richard H. and Beatrice Griffey, Ph.D., Nicholas A. Matwiyoff, Ph.D., Department of Cell Biology, New Mexico University; Edgar Alzner, Ph.D., The Fonar Corporation; Jun Hasegawa, M.S., Asahi Chemical Industry Co., Kanagawa, Japan.

I gratefully acknowledge the invaluable assistance of Holde Muller, Vickie Soufflet, Charlene Levering, Julie Victorian, Linda Toda and the staff of Stanford's Visual Art Services for computer graphics support and the medical graphics staff of Stanford's Office of Instructional Media for their patient work in preparing the graphic illustrations and in manuscript preparation. And I am deeply indebted to Ann Patterson, Diana Schneider, and Mary Rogers for their encouragement and advice in preparing this book.

Finally, I am indebted to James E. Howell, Kreps Professor of Macroeconomics, who was my macroeconomics professor at the Stanford Graduate School of Business and who first introduced me to the macroeconomic approach taken in Chapter 7.

Foreword

In the five years since it was introduced into general clinical practice, magnetic resonance imaging (MRI) has revolutionized the practice of radiology. Not only are the physics of image formation substantially different from those of X-ray, gamma-ray, or ultrasound-based techniques, the determinants of contrast are different as well. Radiologists who completed their residencies prior to five years ago received little formal training in MRI. Thus, these radiologists are now faced with learning this new imaging technique on their own. Furthermore, they see MRI advancing rapidly into new territory, moving from the early neurologic applications into new regions heretofore within the domain of traditional radiology, e.g., arthrography of the knee. These radiologists must now either learn the most complex imaging technique ever devised, or be forever relegated to the backrooms where they can continue to read plain films and perform barium enemas. It is not that these more experienced physicians do not want to learn MRI; it is just that it is very difficult to assimilate the new material by reading the peer-reviewed literature or by attending a conference.

Unfortunately, most of us do not have the background to assimilate new material at the rate it is dispensed at most MR courses. While textbooks have historically allowed us to learn at our own pace, even textbooks can be intimidating. The basic is often interwoven with the detailed, in a confusing manner for those attempting an overall understanding of MRI. Thus, there is a great need for a text which can lead us through the basics. This is such a text.

The best teacher of a new technique is not necessarily one who is already an "expert". Ideally, we learn best from someone whose background is similar to our own, but from one who has put the time and energy into understanding the basics and who can, therefore, explain it "on our level". Stuart Young has, in fact, accomplished this goal. While he is widely known in academic circles for his expertise in chest radiology and medical economics, he is also known as someone who can take difficult concepts from a field outside his own area of expertise and distill the essence of those concepts. This is exactly what he has done with both editions of this book.

The second edition represents a major improvement on the first (which was entirely adequate for its time). Dr. Young has retained the basic aspects of NMR in general and MRI in particular, while adding basic explanations of topics of current interest as well. These include discussions of the new fast scanning techniques, new flow imaging methods ("MR angiography"), as well as discussions of new developments in the technology of superconductors and medical economics. (On this last

xiii

topic, he is particularly well-qualified, having received his MBA from Stanford Business School in the interval between the first and second editions.)

In summary, I heartily recommend this book to anyone who has wanted to learn the basics of MRI, but who has previously been intimidated by the admittedly difficult technology. Dr. Young has done an excellent job of translating the scientific double-talk so often associated with explanations of MRI into a form which is readily understandable by physicians. Radiologists who take the time and effort to read this book will not be disappointed.

William G. Bradley, M.D., Ph.D.
Huntington Medical Research Institutes
Pasadena, California

Contents

Chapter 1

Nuclear Magnetic Resonance: The Clinical Potential

Magnetic resonance imaging (MRI) is established as an important modality in medical practice. The information density in the nuclear magnetic resonance (NMR) signal is greater than that available from an imaging modality such as computed tomography (X-ray CT) because the magnetic resonance (MR) signal is based on five separate components: density of the nuclear species (usually hydrogen, which is composed of a single proton, ^{1}H); two relaxation times (T_1 and T_2); a phenomenon called chemical shift that enables separate fat and water images to be obtained; and motion or flow. An X-ray CT image, by comparison, is based mainly on X-ray photon interaction with tissue electrons (predominantly coherent scatter and photoelectric effect). The information available from MR images will, in all likelihood, be further enriched when other nuclear species, such as phosphorus and carbon, can be scanned in clinical NMR scanners. The signals from nuclear species other than ^{1}H are low, and therefore the likely format will be to screen these complex data bases using computers and to superimpose phosphorus or carbon images or spectra on hydrogen-density images (anatomic images) either by color tinting of the hydrogen image or by superimposing a black-dot-distribution format similar to that used in autoradiography. Another aspect of NMR imaging that will encourage its clinical utilization is that MRI does not use ionizing radiation and thus is free of the potential hazards of X-rays.

The principles of NMR were first described in 1946, and MRI has been used since 1973. MRI has already been shown to be clearly superior to other competitive imaging modalities (e.g., CT scanning and ultrasound) in certain specific situations. MR images are free of the high-intensity artifacts produced in CT scans by sharp dense bone or metallic surgical clips (e.g., over-range artifacts). Clinically unstable patients and patients on life-support systems are difficult to evaluate with MRI, but MRI is the imaging modality of choice for diagnosing neurological conditions such as multiple sclerosis. By selecting the proper MRI techniques, areas of edema, hemorrhage, and flowing blood, which are difficult to distinguish using X-ray CT, can be resolved using MRI.

The clinical applications of MRI are expanding rapidly. All parts of the anatomy, from the head to the extremities (Figs. 1.1 to 1.3), are currently evaluated with

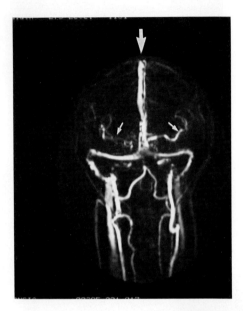

FIG. 1.1. A small-tip-angle/gradient-recalled echo MRI vascular imaging sequence of the head using a coronal projection technique. Both venous and arterial vascular structures are seen as high-intensity signals, and static tissue has been suppressed. The superior sagittal sinus (*large arrow*) and left and right middle cerebral arteries (*small arrows*) are marked. The sigmoid sinuses are seen bilaterally as acutely bending structures just below the middle cerebral arteries. The carotid arteries and venous structures of the neck overlap. The vertebral arteries are seen joining to form the basilar artery, which is seen *en face* just below the inferior extent of the cerebral sagittal sinus. (Courtesy of the General Electric Co.)

FIG. 1.2. A coronal MRI study through the volar aspect of the right hand in a normal patient. This somewhat T_1-weighted partial saturation spin echo (PSSE) sequence (TR/TE = 600/20) provides a good anatomic view of the carpal tunnel. The tubercle (crest) of the trapezium or great multangular (*largest white arrow*), the pisiform (*middle-size white arrow*), and the hook of the hamate (*smallest white arrow*) are indicated. Also identified are the first metacarpal and the proximal phalanx of the fifth digit (little finger)(1&5). The tendons of the carpal tunnel are linear black structures between the marrow or high-intensity signal of these bones. The first through the fifth tendons of the flexor digitorum profundus are seen passing through the carpal tunnel and then fanning out toward their respective digits.

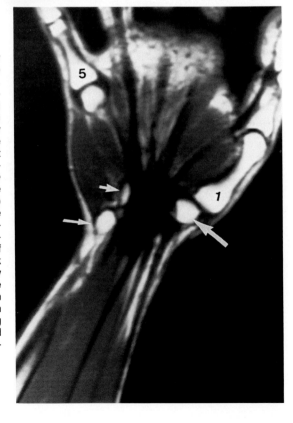

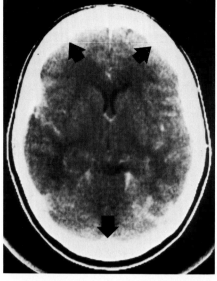

A

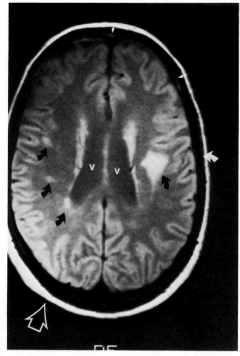

B

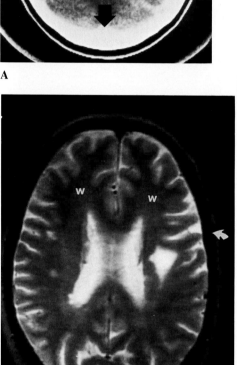

C

FIG. 1.3. A normal CT scan (**A**) for comparison with two axial images from a 61-year-old female patient with recent onset of symptoms of multiple sclerosis (**B** & **C**, 2,000/40/80) and sagittal and coronal images from a normal individual with some T_1 weighting (600/20). This sequence illustrates some of the differences between MRI and CT and some of the advantages of MRI over CT. Note that on the X-ray CT scan the bone of the skull is a dense white outer ring (*black arrows*), and little of the subcutaneous tissue is visualized, whereas on the MR images the bone is noted by its appearance as a black density around the brain (*curved white arrows*), and the subcutaneous fat is seen as a dense white circumferential ring (*open white arrow*) on balanced and T_1-weighted images (**B, D,** and **E**, respectively). With T_2 weighting (**C**), there is a marked decrease in the intensity of the signal emanating from the subcutaneous fat (*open white arrow*). Some MR signal is obtained from the central portion of the bony skull. This signal emanates from the fat contained in the bone marrow (*short arrows*). By changing the MR imaging sequence, different features of the tissue can be elucidated. For example, the cerebrospinal fluid (V) is seen as a low-intensity tissue on T_1-weighted and balanced images (**C, D,** & **E**), whereas it is seen as a high-intensity signal on a more T_2-weighted image (**C**).

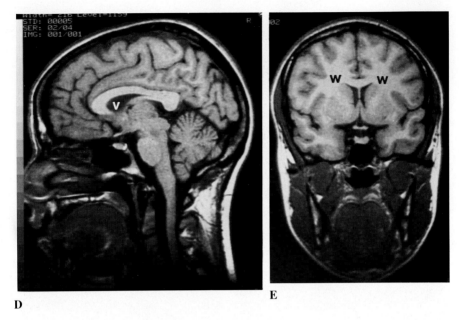

D

E

FIG. 1.3. (*continued*). White matter is seen as a signal of relatively low intensity (W) on balanced and more T_2-weighted images, whereas on T_1-weighted images (**D** & **E**) it is seen as a signal of relatively high intensity, of greater intensity than surrounding gray matter. Note the corpus callosum suspended between the two W's on the coronal image (**E**). MRI is the study of choice for evaluating patients with multiple sclerosis. In this patient (**B** & **C**), the only positive finding was an IgG synthesis rate that was 10 times normal at the time of onset of some vague clinical symptoms. The current study reveals multiple plaques of multiple sclerosis located throughout the white matter (*curved black arrows*). In addition to providing the ability to further identify tissues on the basis of their nuclear density and T_1 and T_2 characteristics by manipulating the imaging sequences, MRI has an advantage over conventional CT scanning in that the three orthogonal views are readily obtainable using conventional imaging sequences, and oblique scanning is also now available.

MRI, often as the modality of choice. Vascular imaging has shown promising results with both arteries and veins (Fig. 1.1).

Image quality in MRI is excellent. With the use of surface coils and more sensitive head and body coils, structures such as the cranial nerves (Fig. 1.4), small joints, and temporomandibular joint (Fig. 1.5) can be effectively evaluated. The field of view for MRI is also expanding, and whole-body screening for metastatic disease and other total-body processes is now a reality (Fig. 1.6).

Significant advances have been made in MRI evaluation of the vertebral column and spinal cord. Much of the utility of MRI in this anatomic area has been related to the development of gating and fast scanning techniques (Fig. 1.7). The NMR signal void related to rapidly flowing blood has made MRI useful for evaluating blood vessels and pathological conditions involving the mediastinum. The low-intensity signal from flowing blood and the high-intensity signal from mediastinal

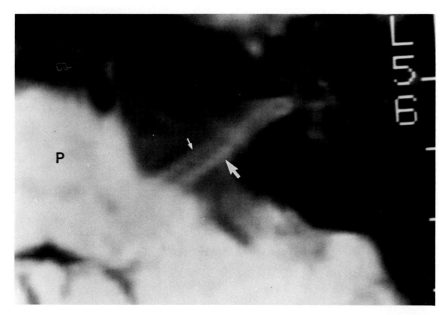

FIG. 1.4. An axial MRI study of a normal volunteer (800/20) revealing normal cranial nerve anatomy of the seventh (*small arrow*) and eighth (*large arrow*) vestibulocochlear nerves emanating from the pons (P). The nerve can be followed through its course in the internal auditory canal. The cochlea and vestibular apparatus are indistinctly seen in this image.

fat contrast sharply with the intermediate-intensity signal from metastases or primary neoplasms of the mediastinum and hilum (Fig. 1.8). This flow-void phenomenon has also been useful in evaluating normal and pathological conditions in the brain (Figs. 1.9 and 1.10). MRI scanning of the abdomen and pelvis is experiencing rapid advances. However, technical problems in controlling cardiovascular and respiratory motion, as well as the availability of competing cost-effective modalities such as CT, ultrasound, angiography, and barium studies, have, in comparison with neurological applications, slowed these MRI applications. Nevertheless, uses of MRI for diagnostic body scanning are expanding rapidly (Figs. 1.11 and 1.12).

The tempo of change in MRI in medicine has been accelerating and continues to accelerate at a bewildering rate, even for those whose expertise is primarily in the imaging sciences. Developments and applications of MRI are expanding more rapidly than in other imaging techniques such as CT, partly because the information obtained with MRI is based on the biochemistry of the tissue. Anatomic delineation occurs as a consequence of the characteristic biochemical nature of the individual organ. Understanding and effectively using the *in vivo* biochemical information made available for the first time by MRI are exciting and demanding challenges. We are only at the threshold of this important development in medical science.

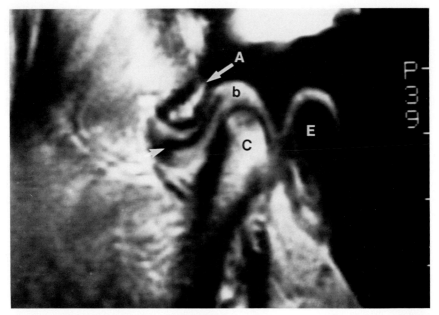

A

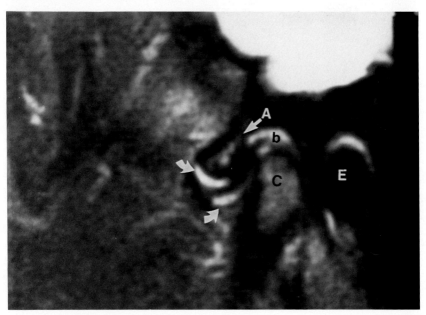

B

FIG. 1.5. Closed-mouth (**A** & **B,** 2,000/20/80) and open-mouth (**C** & **D,** 2,000/20/80) sagittal MRI studies using a proton surface coil in a patient with temporomandibular joint pain and a clinical click. The meniscus (*white arrow,* A) is seen to be reduced on the open-mouth view behind the condyle (C), and there are associated superior and inferior effusions (*curved white arrows*). This patient was also undergoing splint therapy, and with the splint in place (not shown) the meniscus was not reduced and was entrapped anterior to the condyle (C).

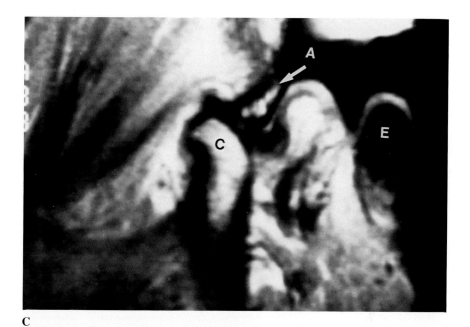

C

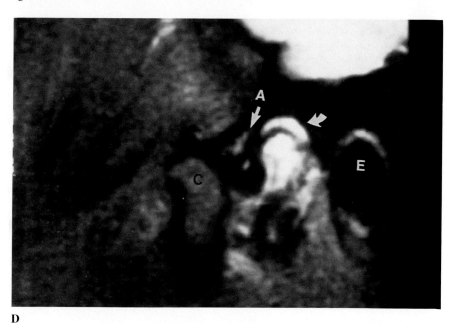

D

FIG. 1.5. *(continued).* In splint therapy, it is important for the splint to be placed after reduction of the meniscus; otherwise, further inflammation and tension on the meniscus and bilaminar zone occur. Therapy was adjusted during this series of MR images. Marrow is seen as a high-intensity signal in the articular eminens (A), the condyle of the mandible (C), and surrounding the external auditory canal (E). The bilaminar zone (b) is also marked.

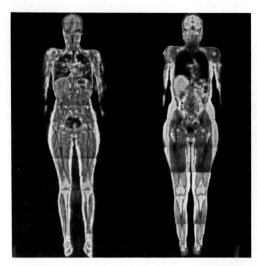

FIG. 1.6. Two coronal whole-body MRI studies obtained using a digitally driven air-suspension couch, with 450 contiguous axial slices requiring an acquisition time of 4.2 min and a full-body scan time of 8.4 min (150/7; 0.3-T permanent magnet). (Courtesy of the Fonar Corporation.)

FIG. 1.7. Three sagittal MRI studies of (**A**) a normal cervical vertebral column, (**B**) a traumatic herniation of the nucleus (*white arrow*) in the midthoracic vertebral column, and (**C**) a large herniation in the L4-5 lumbar vertebral column (*white arrows*). Note the excellent anatomic detail, although there is some signal fall-off due to the posteriorly placed surface coil, noted mostly in images **A** and **C.** The basis vertebral veins (*black arrows*) are noted in **B.** Sagittal imaging has greatly improved the diagnostic potential of MRI in conjunction with gated and fast scanning techniques.

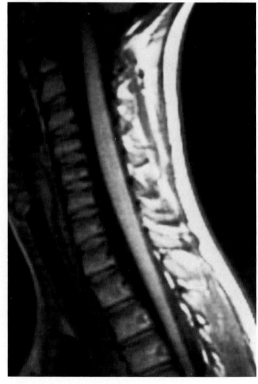

A

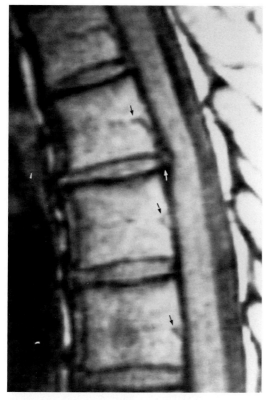

B

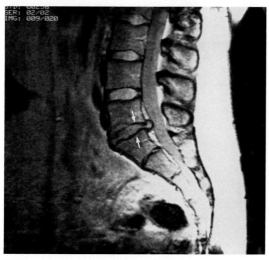

C

FIG. 1.7. (*Continued*). **B** and **C.**

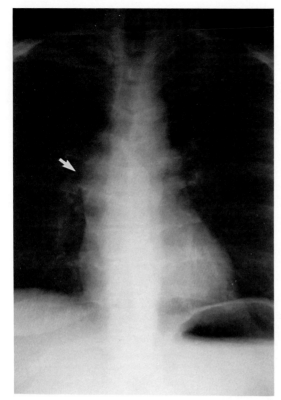

FIG. 1.8. PA-plane radiograph of the chest (**A**) and axial MRI study (**B**, 800/20) in a patient with a previously diagnosed lymphoma and an increase in the right mediastinal contour on a recent chest X-ray (*white arrow*). The MR image reveals that this was due to increased fat deposition in the mediastinum in this patient, who was on steroid therapy. Identified are the ascending and descending (A) aorta, main pulmonary artery (P), the proximal portion of the right main pulmonary artery, the superior vena cava (S), the left (L) and right (R) main-stem bronchi, and the azygos vein emptying into the superior vena cava (*arrow*). The mediastinal fat is seen enveloping the anterior mediastinum, subcarinal area, and the left main-stem bronchus (*bullets*). Also note the cerebrospinal fluid flow artifact posterior and lateral to the spinal cord.

A

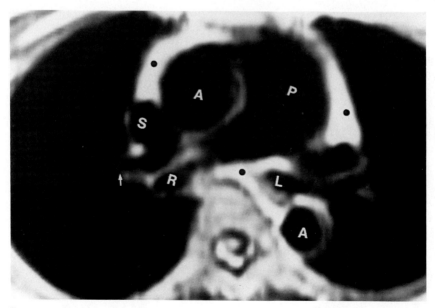

B

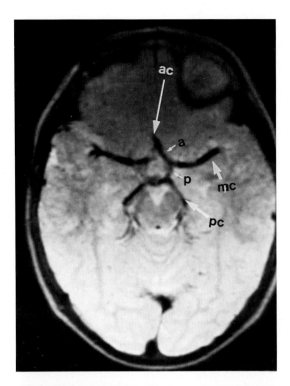

FIG. 1.9. Although there is an inhomogeneity artifact (note the signal falloff from posterior to anterior) in this axial MRI study of a normal 3-year-old brain, the flow void provides excellent anatomic detail of the circle of Willis. Indicated are the anterior, middle, and posterior cerebral arteries (ac, mc, pc) and the anterior and posterior communicating arteries (a, p). The basilar artery is seen as a slight enlargement at the origin of the two posterior cerebral arteries.

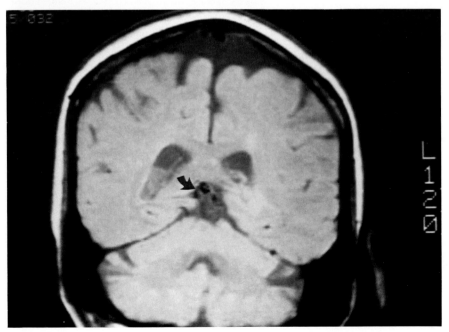

A

FIG. 1.10. Legend on page 12.

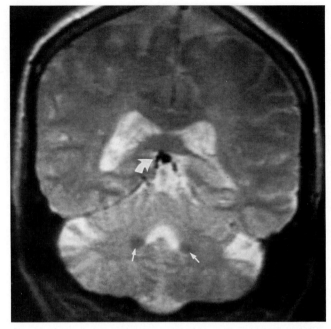

B

FIG. 1.10. Two coronal images (1,500/40/80) in a patient with an arteriovenous malformation (*curved arrows*). Note also that on the more T_2-weighted image (**B**) the dentate nuclei are seen (*small white arrows*) at either end of the higher-intensity cerebrospinal fluid in the fourth ventricle. The flow void, in combination with the increased intensity of the cerebrospinal fluid, provides excellent anatomic detail of the exact location of the arteriovenous malformation in this patient.

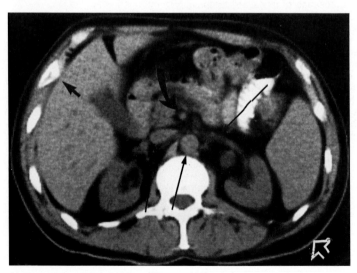

A

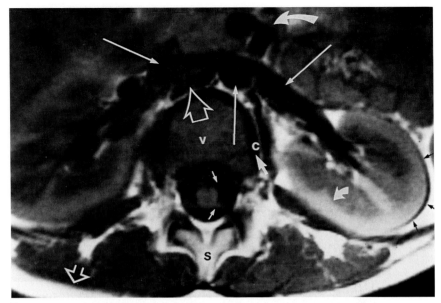

B

FIG. 1.11. Normal X-ray CT scan (**A**) and normal MR image (**B**) obtained at the level of the left renal vein. As in the previous comparisons with CT scans, note the reversal in gray-scale density for bone, which is white on X-ray CT scans (**A,** *short black arrow*) and may appear on MRI scans as a low-intensity signal for cortical bone (c, above *white arrow*); intermediate intensity may be seen, depending on the amount of bone marrow present, as in the vertebral body (v); a high-density signal is seen if a considerable amount of fatty marrow is contained (s, marrow contained in the dorsal spine of a lower thoracic vertebra). Subcutaneous fat also demonstrates reversed signal intensities for CT and MRI (*open arrowheads*). Another useful difference between X-ray CT and MRI illustrated by these body sections is the absence of signal from rapidly moving blood within blood vessels in the MR image, as opposed to the soft-tissue density seen on the X-ray CT scans. This phenomenon is seen in the inferior vena cava, aorta, and left renal vein (*long arrows*). Also noted is the right renal artery (*open arrowhead*, **B**) taking it's origin from the aorta. The superior mesenteric artery and vein are also demonstrated (*large curved arrows*). Additional information is provided from the MRI study regarding the kidney as the corticomedullary junction is sharply defined, even without the use of intravenous contrast material (*curved white arrow*). The dorsal and ventral nerve roots emanating from the spinal cord are seen on the MR image (*small white arrows*), but not the CT scan. The signal falloff between the left kidney and right kidney is an artifact due to magnetic inhomogeneity within the system (**B**) (1.5 T; 800/20; 256 × 256 matrix; 5-mm slice thickness; two excitations; 20% skip between slices). Also note chemical-shift artifact around the left kidney (*small black arrows*) seen laterally as a low-intensity curvilinear structure.

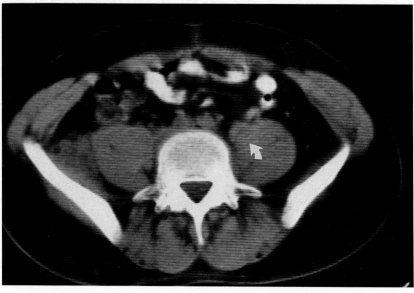

A

FIG. 1.12.   Axial CT (**A**) and two coronal MRI studies (**B & C,** 1,500/40 and 800/20, respectively) in a patient with previously treated Hodgkin's disease of the right quadriceps femoris and surrounding tissue. The patient was referred for follow-up evaluation. CT findings were grossly normal. The left psoas was seen to be infiltrated with Hodgkin's disease on the MRI medially (*curved white arrow*). A soft-tissue density lateral to the right psoas was believed to have been an unopacified loop of bowel on CT. MRI evaluation revealed this area to be a complex structure (*angled white arrow*) that later was found to be a recurrence of Hodgkin's disease between the right psoas and iliacus muscles (P, I). The more T$_1$-weighted image revealed previously undiagnosed benign prostatic hypertrophy in this relatively young 24-year-old male (C, *arrow*). There was fatty-marrow replacement of the right femur (c). The patient had had previous irradiation in this area related to therapy for surrounding Hodgkin's disease.

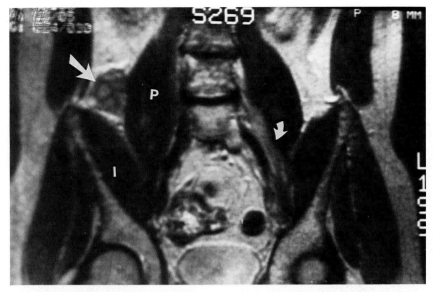

B

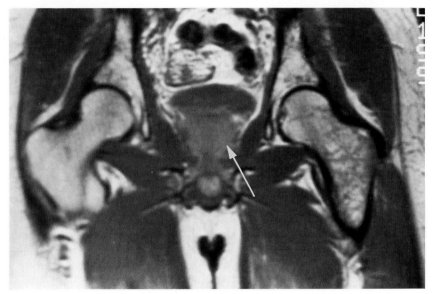

C

FIG. 1.12. (*continued*).

HOW TO USE THIS BOOK

For many imaging specialists who have only recently become familiar with the principles, techniques, normal anatomic findings, and artifacts encountered with ultrasound, CT, and digital imaging, the prospect of learning the underlying physical principles and clinical applications of an entirely new technology is not taken lightly. CT and ultrasound can be used fairly effectively without an extensive understanding of radiation physics and digital image-reconstruction techniques. MRI is much more complex, and images can provide different information depending on many interacting aspects of the imaging sequence and the tissue being evaluated. MRI will continue to be an increasingly important tool for medical diagnosis and treatment evaluation and, in all likelihood, will at some point exceed the capacity of CT scanning as a diagnostic modality. Consequently, to use these techniques effectively, the clinician is obliged to understand the basics of NMR imaging, particularly as they relate to clinical interpretation.

MRI may seem fairly simple at first, because many of the images look like CT or ultrasound scans. MRI may seem exceptionally complex on further consideration. However, it is the objective of this book to develop each principle and concept in NMR as if composing a fugue, using many examples from common experience. Each principle will be discussed—first, by analogy with sound waves, and second by analogy with magnetic compass needles. Finally, these analogies will be used as a foundation for more complex explanations of NMR physics, MRI principles, and image interpretation.

Readers of this book will have varying degrees of knowledge of NMR. Many will not need all of the fundamental analogies presented here and may wish to read the more advanced MRI explanations and clinical material. The redundancies in the analogies are intentional. I have introduced principles to provide a foundation and, subsequently, reiterated and built on them in the hope that concepts not completely comprehensible in one form of imagery will be understandable in another. An MRI quiz is included at the end of this book for those who may wish to evaluate their level of understanding and earmark sections to be included in a quick subject review. Images have been selected to illustrate the topics discussed in the chapter on gray-scale determinants in MRI, as well as to illustrate clinical applications.

Finally, although there are sections devoted to MRI artifacts and an atlas of normal anatomy, both normal anatomy and artifacts are extensively illustrated throughout the book. Illustrations are annotated to indicate the images in a series that have more, "relative", T_1-weighting or T_2-weighting than other comparison images. Readers should be aware that absolute T_1-weighting and T_2-weighting statements, as commonly used, are misleading and overly simplified, since all tissues have a unique combinations of spin density, relaxation times, flow/motion, and chemical shift effects. Thus any given pulsing sequence may have significantly different regional signal component contributions in any one given scan.

Chapter 2

Magnetic Resonance Imaging Systems

MAGNETS

There are two general types of magnets: permanent magnets and electromagnets, which are created by electric current. The simplest example of a permanent magnet is the bar magnet. MRI permanent-magnet systems are constructed of bricks of permanently magnetized material, variably composed of iron, neodymium, boron, etc. Permanent magnets provide excellent image quality (see Fig. 1.6), and their expenses involving operation and site preparation are low. Permanent magnets have some drawbacks in that they are sensitive to changes in temperature and are very heavy, and surface scratches or bits of metal will alter the homogeneity of the magnetic field. Nevertheless, permanent-magnet systems do not have many of the problems that arise with superconducting or resistive magnets. With permanent magnets there is no potential for quenching, nor any special power requirements. There is a minimal fringe field and a limited missile effect, so site selection is much less difficult. There are no costly cryogenic expenses, and there are no moving parts, except for the motorized patient cot. Thus, the chief advantages of permanent magnets are low maintenance costs and little cost for site preparation.

There are two types of resistive magnets that use electric current, depending on the type of core: iron-core and air-core. An iron-core magnet consists of a large central C- or H-shaped block of iron, with multiple turns of a resistive conductor (usually copper or aluminum) wrapped around it. Such wires may also be suspended in space, creating a so-called air-core magnet. High-quality diagnostic imaging is currently being performed with resistive systems (see Fig. 6.24). In superconducting imaging systems (see images, Fig. 1.3) the current-carrying conductors are made of niobium-titanium (NbTi) embedded in a copper matrix. The conductor is submerged in liquid helium, which in turn is surrounded by a vacuum; there is a subsequent layer of liquid nitrogen, then another vacuum, and finally insulation. The copper matrix for the NbTi conductors protects the system from destruction in case of an accidental quench (i.e., a loss of superconductivity). When running at superconducting temperatures ($4°K$), the copper serves as a heat conductor, but not as an electrical conductor, whereas the NbTi, which has no resistance, conducts the

17

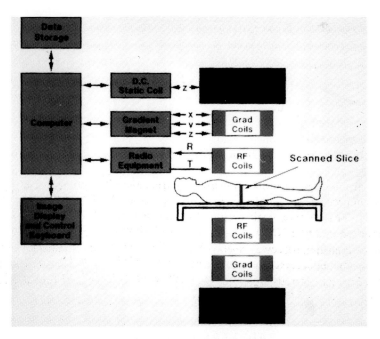

FIG. 2.1. Schematic representation of a typical imaging system showing the six basic MRI subsystems: RF transmitter-receiver coil, magnetic-gradient coil, static external-field magnet, computer, data storage, and display.

current. If the temperature begins to rise, however, the copper quickly becomes the less resistive of the two conductors and safely dissipates the current previously confined to the NbTi conductors, which prevents melting of these wire filaments. New alloys have been developed that are capable of superconducting at around 250°K, and superconduction at higher temperatures seems to be a likely future development. If these elements can be used in clinical imaging, dissemination of MRI systems and their applications will greatly accelerate.

A resistive magnet creates a magnetic field by passing an electric current through a wire wrapped around a core. The larger the current and the greater the number of turns of wire, the greater the magnetic field created. The limit on magnetic field strength appears to be primarily related to the amount of heat that is created by the current as it flows against the resistance of the wire. To create magnetic fields, very large currents are required, e.g., 100 to 150 amperes (A). In addition, the magnet creates sufficient heat that it must be water-cooled (which can require several liters of water per minute). Magnetic fields of 3 to 4 kilogauss (kG) can be obtained with resistive magnets, but at this point, the power consumption, cooling requirements, and bulk (weight) of the magnet appear to limit higher fields with resistive systems. Above 3 kG, the advantages are in favor of the superconducting magnets. The available evidence indicates that images obtained with magnetic fields in excess of 1.5 kG are superior to those obtained below 1.5 kG. At the higher field strengths, the NMR signal strength and signal-to-noise ratio increase, and the imaging time can be decreased. Once the magnet is approximately up to field strength, a super-conducting magnet operates without using any additional electric current. The large power consumption required by resistive magnets is eliminated. The magnetic field can be maintained at a constant strength with high uniformity. Both of these factors are important for improving image detail.

The components for an NMR imaging system are fairly well defined, although undoubtedly there will be modifications to each of these units as time progresses. A large magnet is used to impose a strong external and relatively uniform magnetic field. Within the aperture of the magnet there is a series of current-carrying gradient coils that modify the uniformity of the external field. These gradient coils are used to spatially encode the NMR signal. Next, a transmitter is connected to a radio-frequency transmitter-receiver antenna with which the radio-frequency pulse is broadcast into and received from the sample (or object) being scanned. The image is then amplified, filtered, digitized, and processed by a computer for image recon-struction and display (Fig. 2.1).

RADIO-FREQUENCY COILS

A schematic radio-frequency (RF) coil is shown in Fig. 2.2. The factors involved in its functioning are the inductance, L, the capacitances, C, the resistance, R, and

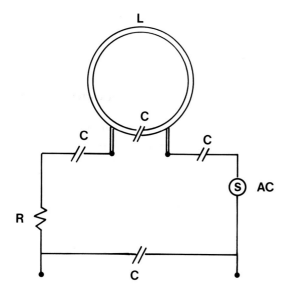

FIG. 2.2. Schematic RF coil represented as a series *LRC* circuit with an AC power source. The circuit inductance, *L*, is determined by the coil geometry. The capacitances, *C*, are adjusted in series to select the resonant frequency and output impedance. The AC power source is used to broadcast RF signals. The MR signal consists of both signal from the precessing nuclei and noise from the system.

an alternating-current (AC) power source. An RF coil can have any shape. The coil is tuned to broadcast or receive a certain frequency by adjusting the capacitances in series. The resistance, R, will depend on the closeness of the spacing between the coil and the patient. The inductance, L, is determined by the geometry of the coil. The inductance increases linearly as the dimensions of the coil are increased. The circular coil is the simplest and often is used in surface-coil design. In the receiving mode, a voltage is recorded from the tissue that alternates at the frequency of rotation of the nuclei (discussed in the next chapter) in the body. The voltage NMR signal represents both the MR signal for the precessing nuclei and the noise in the system.

MRI systems often use a saddle-shaped coil for both transmitting and receiving functions. Large body coils and smaller circumferential head coils are commonly used. Special-purpose coils and paired-coil series are also used in special scanning situations. Surface coils provide an improved signal-to-noise ratio over a limited field of view. Although surface coils can be used for both transmitter and receiver functions, the usual approach is to take advantage of the uniformity of excitation provided by the larger coils (body or head coils) and use the local (surface) coils as receiver elements.

GRADIENT COILS

Gradient coils are used to encode spatial information in the MR signal. They can have many configurations; a schematic version is shown in Fig. 2.3. Gradient coils create opposing magnetic fields because they carry currents in opposite directions. The field from one coil "opposes" the field from the other, creating a net field that is a gradient between the two coils. By independently altering the current in each coil, the steepness of the gradient can be controlled. These gradients are typically on the order of a few G per centimeter, and there is a zero-strength gradient point between the two coils. Gradients can be applied in any of the three orthogonal directions, although other configurations are possible. Eddy currents created in the housing of the scanner (or patient) have been greatly reduced by electrically shielding the gradient coils of the magnet.

STATIC MAGNETIC FIELD

As discussed previously, the static field is produced by either a permanent magnet or an electromagnet. The field should be homogeneous, and higher field strengths offer the possibility of performing imaging with an increased signal-to-noise ratio and better line-width separation (see Chapter 8) when performing *in vivo* spectroscopy. These options come at a certain higher price, but have evolving diagnostic benefits.

A partially constructed superconducting magnet is shown in Fig. 2.4, and a generic magnet configuration is shown in Fig. 2.5.

GRADIENT COILS

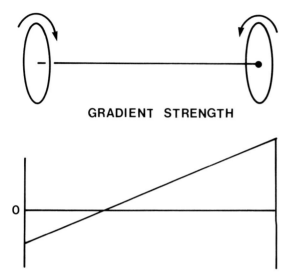

GRADIENT STRENGTH

DISTANCE BETWEEN COILS

FIG. 2.3. Schematic representation of a gradient coil. The coils carry current in opposing directions and are placed in the three orthogonal planes inside the scanner. They are used to encode spatial information in MRI. The magnetic fields from the two coils are in opposition and create a gradient of magnetic field strength between the coils. The zero-gradient point and the steepness of the gradient can be adjusted by independently altering the currents in the coils.

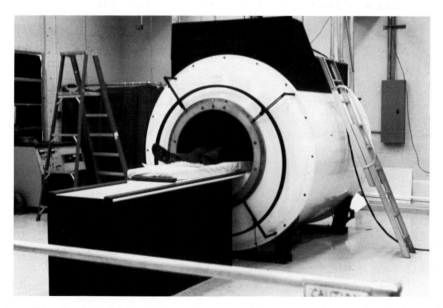

FIG. 2.4. Superconducting magnet being assembled into an MRI system. The helium and nitrogen cryogens are contained in the shell along with the wire for generating the magnetic field. The gradient and RF coil will be placed inside the housing and will be at room temperature.

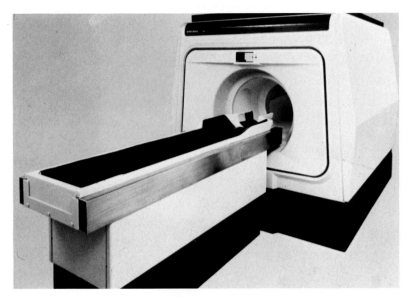

FIG. 2.5.   Generic configuration and appearance of an MRI system after it is assembled.

Chapter 3

Magnetic Resonance: What Is It?

HISTORICAL PERSPECTIVE

The principles of NMR were originally described in 1946 by Bloch at Stanford, for liquids, and by Purcell at Harvard, for solids. In 1952 they received the Nobel Prize for their observations. In 1951, Gabillard first noted that spatial localization appeared to be possible with NMR. The primary impetus for development of the current generation of imaging techniques was a publication by Lauterbur in *Nature* in 1973 regarding a spatial coding and back-projection reconstruction technique in NMR that he termed *zeugmatography*. In 1975, EMI began prototype development of a commercial MR imager, and subsequently there was an explosion of research and development in MRI techniques.

As discussed previously, the NMR signal is based on a complex set of tissue parameters including hydrogen density and two separate relaxation times (T_1 and T_2). Because it takes a finite time to register the signal from the excited hydrogen nuclei, no NMR signal is recorded from fast-moving nuclei. In other words, the technique is very sensitive to motion and flow. By using these four parameters for ^1H, a wealth of clinical information is potentially available from NMR studies. Hydrogen nuclei produce different signals depending on the type of tissue being imaged. Images based on either fat or water protons can be obtained using this phenomenon, called chemical shift. These five components of the hydrogen signal are in contrast with the signal obtained with transmission X-ray CT, for example, in which the information is largely based on a physical characteristic: X-ray interaction with tissue electrons and tissue electron density and atomic number.

Briefly, MRI is a way of making pictures of the body that look somewhat like CT scans. Atoms in the body can act like tiny bar magnets, with a north pole and a south pole. When an external magnetic field is applied across a part of the body, each little magnet lines up with the external magnetic field. If a radio wave (RF wave) is then broadcast into the tissue, some of the magnets are induced by the energy from the radio wave to tilt over. The radio wave is then turned off, and subsequently the magnets transmit or rebroadcast a signal of the same frequency as the original RF wave. A receiver antenna inside the scanner picks up the signal from the atomic magnets, and a computer can process the signal and make a picture (image) from the signal.

RADIO WAVES AND THE ELECTROMAGNETIC SPECTRUM

An understanding of MRI requires a fundamental grasp of the concepts of electromagnetic waves, magnetism, and resonance. Radio waves make up one subdivision of electromagnetic waves. One way of conceptualizing an electromagnetic wave is as a waveform with its electric and magnetic components perpendicular to each other and perpendicular to the line of the wave's propagation. This is an important consideration to remember in MRI because it is the magnetic component of the electromagnetic wave that interacts with the magnetic field of the tissue protons. The effect of this interaction will be perpendicular to the line of propagation of the electromagnetic wave, or, in this case, the RF wave. Thus, the directionality of the RF pulse used to irradiate tissue in an NMR scanner is critical, because in MRI it is very important to change the magnetic vector in the tissue in various specific ways. For now, however, it is sufficient to recall that the magnetic force acts perpendicular to the line of propagation of the radio wave (Figs. 3.1 and 3.2).

Electromagnetic waves are characterized by (a) frequency, or the number of cycles per second (1 cps = 1 hertz, Hz), (b) energy (electron volts), and (c) wavelength (meters). The relationship among frequency, energy, and wavelength for electromagnetic waves is such that energy and wavelength are inversely related. In understanding MRI it is helpful to remember this direct association among electromagnetic wave energy, increasing frequency, and decreasing wavelength.

Within the electromagnetic spectrum, visible light is the portion with which we are most familiar. The electromagnetic spectrum is a continuum of waves with both electronic and magnetic properties. For medical diagnosis in the human body, visible light is indeed a useful portion of the electromagnetic spectrum, because many diseases have surface manifestations. However, visible light is not useful when trying to obtain images from inside the human body. In this regard, radiologists have traditionally used the narrow spectrum of X-rays of fairly high energy (Fig.

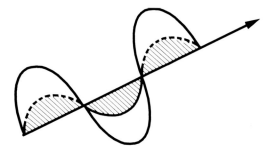

FIG. 3.1. Radio waves are a form of electromagnetic radiation with electric and magnetic components that are perpendicular to the line of the propagation, indicated by the central vector (*arrow*) in this figure. Thus, the magnetic interaction in NMR imaging is perpendicular to the line of propagation of the radio waves.

ELECTROMAGNETIC WAVES

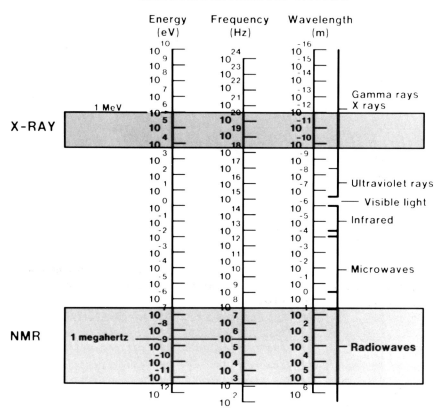

FIG. 3.2. The electromagnetic spectrum is actually a continuum of electromagnetic waves. X-rays, visible light, and radio waves are useful in medical diagnosis; however, only X-rays and, more recently, radio waves in conjunction with NMR imaging have been harnessed to noninvasively image inside the body.

3.2) to image internal organs of the body and to make the familiar black-and-white X-ray films of the bones and other internal organs. Now, with the development of MRI, that portion of the electromagnetic spectrum that consists of radio waves appears to provide a second useful source of energy with which we can noninvasively study internal organs.

MAGNETS AND MAGNETIC CONCEPTS

A magnet is any piece of iron, steel, or, originally, magnetite (lodestone) that has the property of attracting iron, steel, etc. This property may be naturally present or may be artificially induced by passing an electric current through a coil of wire wrapped around the metal. Magnetic force is the force with which a magnet attracts a piece of iron or steel. Similarly, a magnetic field is the space around the magnet in which its magnetic force is appreciable or measurable.

The gauss (G) is the most common unit for measuring magnetic field strength; 1 G is the measured magnetic field strength at 1 cm from a straight wire carrying a current of 5 A. Generally speaking, the field strengths used in MRI are on the order of thousands of gauss. Magnetic fields usually are measured in kilogauss (1,000 G = 1 kG) or tesla (T), where 1 T = 10 kG. The gauss is named for Karl Friedrich Gauss (1777–1855), a German mathematician who made the first absolute measurement of the geomagnetic field of the earth on May 26, 1832. He devoted much of his scientific life to standardizing and quantifying the measurement of magnetic fields. The tesla is named for Nikola Tesla (1857–1943), and Austrian-born electrician who came to the United States in 1884 and was one of the first to develop practical applications of the principle of the rotating magnetic field.

Magnetic Fields

We are all familiar with the generation of magnetic fields and magnetic moments. For example, the north and south magnetic poles of the earth are produced by the magnetohydrodynamic action of the earth's core. The spinning of the earth creates an angular magnetic moment that results in the earth's magnetic field, and in the same manner, a magnetic field is produced by charged nuclear particles spinning within body tissues. This principle is extremely important in MRI. An important consideration regarding the earth's magnetic field is that its magnetic field strength is not uniform, but rather weaker at the equator (approximately 0.3 G) than at the north pole (approximately 0.7 G). Thus, there is a gradient in the earth's magnetic field, and by measuring that gradient we can determine whether we are at the equator or at the pole or anywhere in between (Fig. 3.3). In a similar manner, gradient magnetic fields are used in MRI to determine spatial localization within tissues.

Any object that possesses charge and velocity will create a magnetic field. Any positively or negatively charged body moving linearly has a magnetic field that is perpendicular to it, the so-called linear magnetic moment. However, a charged body

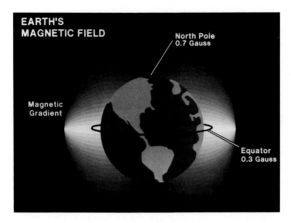

FIG. 3.3. The magnetic field of the earth is one example of angular magnetic moment produced by the rotation of the earth on its axis. The magnetic field is somewhat stronger at the north and south poles than it is at the equator, and by knowing this relationship and the field strength at any given point, one can determine one's latitude on the earth's surface.

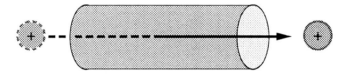

Angular Magnetic Moment

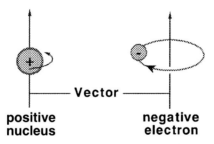

FIG. 3.4. Moving charged particles create a magnetic field called a magnetic moment. Charged particles moving in a linear fashion create a circular magnetic field perpendicular to the line of movement, whereas charged particles that are spinning create an angular magnetic moment whose vector is perpendicular to the rotation of the small charged particles.

that is spinning will produce an angular magnetic vector perpendicular to the rotational axis (Fig. 3.4).

In this book we are concerned primarily with the atomic nucleus in a tissue as the component to be exploited in imaging, and we shall use the earth to provide an analogy for the atomic nucleus in order to help explain the imaging process. Comparing the angular magnetic moment of the earth with the angular magnetic moment

EARTH
MAGNETIC MOMENT

NUCLEAR
MAGNETIC MOMENT

PROTON

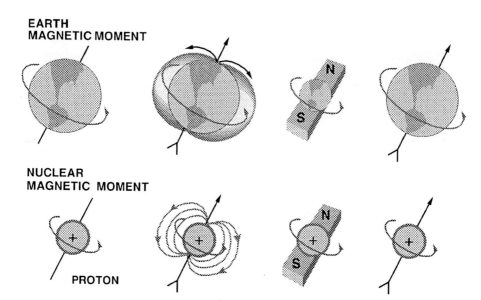

FIG. 3.5. In NMR imaging, the hydrogen nucleus, which is composed of a single proton, and its magnetic field can be compared with the magnetic field of the earth. Both the earth and the proton nucleus spin on an axis. This rotation generates a magnetic field whose vector is perpendicular to the angle of rotation and causes it to function as if it were a magnet with a north pole and south pole. This magnetic dipole, as it is called, usually is represented by a vector indicating the strength and direction of the net magnetic field.

of the nucleus (in this case, the hydrogen nucleus or proton ^{1}H in tissue) is most useful. Both the earth and the ^{1}H nucleus spin on an axis. This spinning creates a magnetic field around each of these bodies, and the net sum of the magnetic field is perpendicular to the axis of rotation. This magnetic field can be represented as a dipole magnet, or as the magnetic vector indicating direction, and magnitude representing the sum of the entire field strength (Fig. 3.5). Vectors representing the summed forces of many magnetic dipoles of spinning nuclei will be the convention used subsequently in this book. There are many atomic nuclear species that possess net charge and spin and therefore possess small magnetic moments. However, some nuclei do not have net spin and magnetic moment.

The Nature of Spinning Particles

The magnitude of angular magnetic moment depends on both the angular momentum (mass × velocity) and charge. Total angular momentum for an electron depends on both its spin and its orbital angular momentum. The majority of nuclei possess spin, although the angular momentum involved varies from nucleus to nucleus. The simplest nucleus is that of the hydrogen atom, which consists of one particle only, the proton. The proton also has a spin of one-half, designated as S. Another particle that is a constituent of all other nuclei is the neutron; this has a unit mass equal to that of the proton, but no charge, and again a spin of one-half. Thus, if a particular nucleus is composed of protons (P) and neutrons (N), its total mass is P + N, its total charge is + P, and its total spin will be a vector combination of P + N spins, each of magnitude one-half. The atomic mass usually is specified for each nucleus by writing it as a superscript prefix to the nuclear symbol, i.e., ^{12}C, which indicates that the nucleus of carbon has a mass of 12. The nucleus ^{13}C (an isotope of carbon) has 6 protons and 7 neutrons. In MRI it is the unpaired nuclear particles that confer the magnetic moment on the nucleus. Thus, ^{12}C, having equal numbers of protons and neutrons, cannot be magnetized, whereas the isotope ^{13}C is magnetized and can be used in MRI and magnetic resonance spectroscopy (MRS) (see Chapter 8). Each nuclear species, being composed of different numbers of protons and neutrons, will have its own total spin value, and, depending on these values, plus the nuclear charge, there may be a strong nuclear magnetic moment or no moment. Without going into more detail, the following generalizations can be made:

1. Nuclei with both P and N even have zero spin (i.e., ^{4}He, ^{12}C, ^{16}O, etc.)
2. Nuclei with both P and N odd [charge odd, but mass (P + N) even] have integral spin [i.e., ^{2}H, ^{14}N (spin equals 1), ^{10}B (spin equals 3), etc.]
3. Nuclei with odd nuclear mass have one-half integral spin [i.e., ^{1}H, ^{15}N (spin = 1/2), ^{17}O (spin = 5/2), etc.]

Electron Paramagnetic Resonance

Previously we have considered the resonance conditions under which spinning particles can interact with electromagnetic radiation (RF). We have heretofore considered this interaction with nuclear species and referred to it as NMR. If the appropriate radiation (microwave) is broadcast into a tissue, however, unpaired electrons are also capable of induction. The magnetic field required to record this interaction must be very homogeneous, but usually of lower field strength, and this phenomenon is referred to as electron paramagnetic resonance (EPR) or sometimes electron spin resonance (ESR). ESR spectroscopy, which involves recording information from unpaired electrons in a given sample, is a well-established technology, and it may well be possible at some point to spatially encode this information and perform ESR experiments. However, the microwave energy requirement will limit the use of ESR in clinical MRI.

Resonance

Tuning forks are helpful in illustrating resonance. In a familiar experiment from high-school science using two tuning forks, both of which are tuned to the note C, one tuning fork is struck and placed next to the other, and the second tuning fork begins to vibrate and emit the note C. This second tone will continue even if the first tuning fork is removed. The first tuning fork is said to have made the second

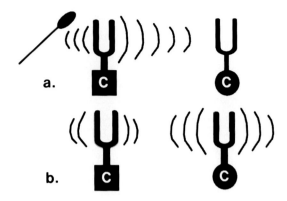

FIG. 3.6. The principle of resonance is probably most easily illustrated with tuning forks. If a tuning fork of a given tone C is struck with a mallet and placed in proximity to another tuning fork of the same tone, the second tuning fork will begin to vibrate and similarly emit the tone C. The second tuning fork can be said to have been made to resonate (produce the tone C) by absorbing energy from the first tuning fork. The resonance of the tone C will persist even if the first tuning fork is removed.

tuning fork resonate. This occurs because they are tuned to the same frequency (note C). Any other frequency will not allow an exchange of energy (Fig. 3.6).

In MRI, the scanner is capable of making the protons spin (discussed in following sections) at exactly the same frequency as the RF pulse being broadcast into the tissue. Some of the protons will be induced to rotate or tip over in a spiral motion. As we shall see, the scanner's antenna can receive MR signals from those protons that have been induced to rotate perpendicular to the antenna, and an image can be made from the information. As with the tuning forks, resonance in NMR is a relationship between matching frequencies. The RF pulse, the spinning frequency of the protons, and the frequency of the MR signal (voltage) induced in the scanner's receiver coil are all the same resonance frequency. Other RF waves do not interact directly within the scanner.

NMR: TERMS REVIEWED

In summary, the fundamental terms of NMR are as follows: *nuclear,* because the magnetic moment used in this technique is provided by spinning charged nuclear particles such as the proton in hydrogen; *magnetic* because the tissue sample is magnetized in an external static magnetic field (this is because of the slight preponderance of parallel over antiparallel protons in the tissue, as discussed in the next sections); *resonance,* because the frequencies of the RF wave and proton spinning must be identical in order to interact and produce the MR signal on which the image is based.

Zeugmatography

Imaging by using NMR was first described as *zeugmatography* by Lauterbur. This term was intended to imply the joining together (*zeugma* is the Greek root meaning "a yoke" or "to yoke together") of the magnetic characteristics of NMR

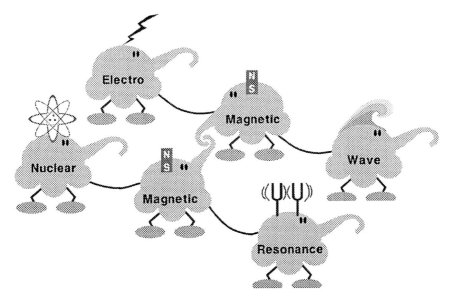

FIG. 3.7. Zeugmatography. The yoke between electromagnetic waves and magnetic nuclei is the interaction in NMR and MRI.

and electromagnetic waves (Fig. 3.7). The electromagnetic waves emitted from a given nuclear species are characteristic in a static magnetic field, permitting the determination of the nuclear species present. Additionally, a gradient magnetic field can be used to assign the nuclei to a position in space within the body.

Net Magnetization

In this section, tissue protons will be discussed briefly as an aid to understanding how they produce a net magnetization of the body. Subsequently the discussion will mainly employ a vector to represent the manipulations of the net magnetization necessary in order to produce an image. It is important to note carefully whether an illustration is using individual protons or vectors representing the summation effect of protons acting in groups, and this point is emphasized in the text where appropriate.

Net magnetization (M) at rest in a weak magnetic field is zero. In body tissues, or any specimen for that matter, before the application of a magnetic field, the magnetic moments of the nuclei making up the tissue are randomly aligned, as shown in Fig. 3.8, and have zero net magnetization ($M = 0$). When an external magnetic field is applied, then after an interval the individual magnetic moments align parallel or antiparallel with the applied net magnetic field, B_0. There is a slight preponderance of nuclei aligned parallel with the magnetic field, and this gives the tissue a net magnetization (M). As an example for ^1H, which has a large magnetic

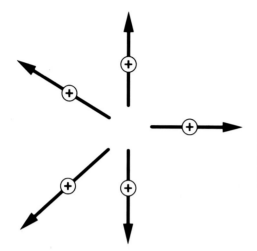

FIG. 3.8. In the absence of an external magnetic field, the magnetic dipoles or vectors of the protons in the tissue align randomly, so that there is no net tissue magnetization.

**TISSUE PROTONS AT REST
NET MAGNETIZATION
(M = O)**

moment in a field of 15 kG, the fractional excess of parallel protons is only about 1×10^{-5} at room temperature. Nevertheless, as small as this slight excess is, it accounts for the small macroscopic net magnetic moment directed parallel with the external magnetic field, and it is this differential that accounts for the NMR signal on which the imaging is based.

Nuclear Spin and Precession

In MRI scanners, the scanning space inside the magnet is divided by three intersecting planes corresponding to the three anatomic planes of the body (e.g., axial, coronal, and sagittal). To avoid having to draw the perpendicular planes in each figure, however, the three planes will be indicated by three intersecting axes (x, y, and z), with the z axis indicating the alignment of the static external magnetic field (Fig. 3.9).

Although it simplifies the discussion to refer to the protons in a magnetic field as being parallel or antiparallel, the protons actually are oriented at an angle to the external field B_z (or B_0), as shown in Fig. 3.10. The two protons are also spinning on their axes (as shown for the two protons illustrated), and this causes the protons to rotate around B_z, as we shall see in a moment.

Another important difference between the parallel and antiparallel protons is that the antiparallel protons are at a slightly higher energy level than the parallel protons. One way to conceptualize this difference in energy states is to consider the different

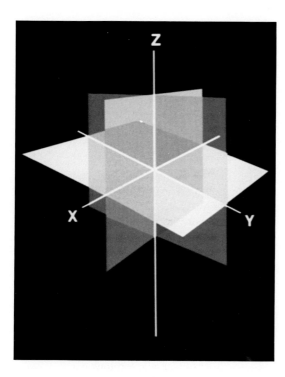

FIG. 3.9. In NMR imaging, the magnetic fields of the scanners are generally oriented in three intersecting perpendicular planes. These three planes can be represented as *x, y,* and *z* axes, and magnetic vectors lying along these axes can be represented as arrows with direction and magnitude. For simplicity throughout the remainder of the text, only the axes will be depicted. However, the reader should recall that these axes are representing three intersecting planes.

FIG. 3.10. Two protons in a magnetic field B_z are said to be parallel and anti-parallel with B_z, although they actually align at a slight angle to B_z. The protons also spin on their respective axes, and, as shown in Fig. 3.11, this spinning action causes the protons to rotate or precess around B_z, and the frequency of rotation is the resonant frequency of the protons and is characteristic of the type of nucleus and the strength of B_z.

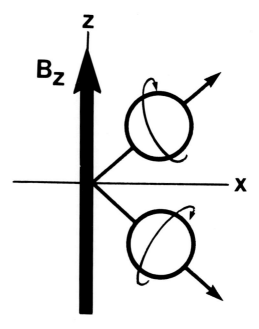

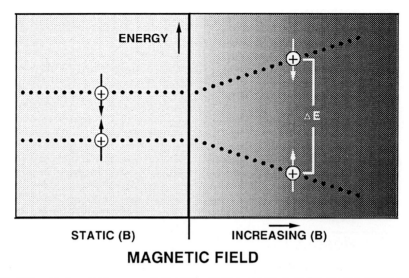

FIG. 3.11. Protons that are parallel with the static magnetic field (*B*) are at a slightly lower energy level than those aligned antiparallel with the static magnetic field. The energy difference between these two states is directly related to the strength of the external magnetic field, such that the energy difference increases with increasing field strength.

energy levels or energy expended by two swimmers, both tied to ropes and attempting to swim toward each other, with one swimming downstream (with the static magnetic field) and the other expending more energy while swimming upstream (against the static magnetic field).

In NMR imaging, the energy differential between the parallel and antiparallel protons is directly proportional to external field strength (Fig. 3.11). The energy differential (ΔE) is given by the equation $\Delta E = (\gamma h/2\pi)B$, where γ is the magnetogyric ratio and B is the external field strength. At this point, the important thing to note about these different energy levels is that the energy differential approximates the thermal energy exchanged between colliding molecules and thus is quite small, i.e., on the order of a 5 to 10 millicalories. At any given field strength, the protons can be induced to "flip" to the higher energy state by RF-wave energy with a frequency matching the rotational frequency (precessional frequency, see next paragraph) of the protons. The energy exchange can occur only at a very specific frequency, and the higher the magnetic field strength, the greater the frequency of resonance and the greater the difference between the energies of the parallel and antiparallel protons.

So far we have represented the magnetic moment of the ensemble of protons in a tissue as being in stable alignment with the external static magnetic field. In actuality, each one of these magnetic moments rotates around the alignment of the static magnetic field in a process called precession. The frequency of rotation is called the precessional frequency (ω) or resonant frequency. By way of analogy,

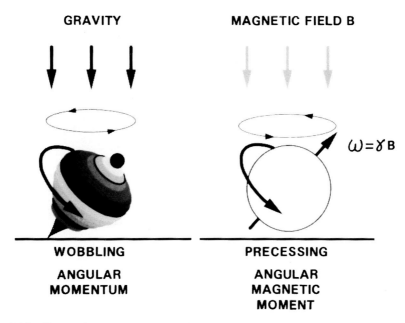

GRAVITY   MAGNETIC FIELD B

$\omega = \gamma B$

WOBBLING   PRECESSING

ANGULAR   ANGULAR
MOMENTUM   MAGNETIC
                            MOMENT

FIG. 3.12. Protons in an external magnetic field do not remain in one position; they wobble or precess around the applied force of the external magnetic field in the same way that a top wobbles in a gravitational field. The frequency (ω) at which the proton precesses is directly related to the strength (B) of the external magnetic field: $\omega = \gamma B$, where γ is the magnetogyric ratio.

the interaction between the proton angular magnetic moment and the external magnetic field is similar to the spinning mass of a top and the earth's gravitation field. The difference is that the competing forces acting on a wobbling top are the earth's static gravitational field trying to push the top down versus the top's angular momentum attempting to keep the top upright (Fig. 3.12). Thus, in a friction-free system, a top spinning on a flat surface possesses a resonant precession or wobble about the direction of the local gravitational field. In a similar manner, a spinning nucleus precesses or wobbles about an applied magnetic field with a resonant angular frequency, determined by a constant (the magnetogyric ratio γ) and the strength of the magnetic field B. Each nuclear species possesses a characteristic value for γ, but ω and B are related by the equation $\omega = \gamma B$. The important relationship in the equation is that the angular frequency for any nuclear species is characteristic and directly proportional to the static magnetic field.

Both the parallel and antiparallel protons undergo precession, as illustrated in Fig. 3.13. The protons are evenly spaced around the circle of precession, and so there is no transverse magnetization. The preponderance of parallel protons, however, confers a net magnetization oriented along B_z. A more graphic representation of the summation of these individual proton vectors is shown in Fig. 3.14. M is the net magnetization vector oriented along the z axis.

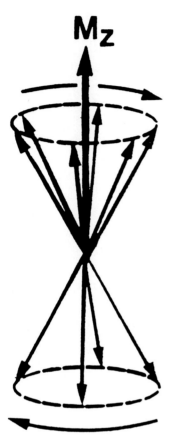

FIG. 3.13. The spinning of the protons around their axes in an external magnetic field causes both the parallel and antiparallel protons to precess or rotate around the external magnetic field. The protons are equally spaced in the precessional orbit, and so there is no transverse (transverse to z) magnetization. However, the slight preponderance of the parallel nuclei confers a net magnetization M_z. For simplification, henceforth in this text, explanations will try to utilize only the net-magnetic-vector display. It is important to bear in mind that during all imaging sequences, all nuclei spin and precess continuously in the same direction. Those figures in the literature displaying protons moving in a reverse rotation are using a rotating frame of reverence and demonstrating a relative motion. The precessional motion also dictates that when protons are inverted or moved, they prescribe a spiraling motion about the axis to achieve their new position. For simplification, the figures in this text will not illustrate the spiraling proton motion during excitation sequences.

FIG. 3.14. This type of display of parallel and antiparallel protons helps to illustrate the net tissue magnetization result of parallel and antiparallel protons. Protons in an external magnetic field (B) align either parallel or antiparallel with the external field, and the nature of this alignment is such that slightly greater numbers are aligned parallel with the external field, which in turn confers a net magnetization of the sample or tissue (M).

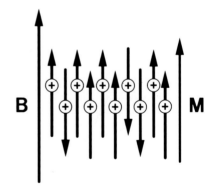

The NMR Signal

Before moving forward to a discussion of the techniques used in imaging with NMR, let us consider in a little more detail the nature of the NMR signal itself. If we review another high-school physics experiment in which a bar magnet is moved perpendicular to a coil with a voltmeter on it, we see that a current is induced. Similarly, if we represent the bar magnet as a vector with direction and magnitude, then as that magnetic vector sweeps past a metal coil, a current will be induced that can be measured (Fig. 3.15). In MRI, the RF signal used to produce the images is recorded in the receiver antenna as the net magnetization vector sweeps past it. The vector sweeps past the coil according to its precessional frequency. For the purposes of explanation, it is sometimes easier to think in terms of a voltage induced in a coil rather than the RF signal recorded in a receiver antenna. But the reader should bear in mind that in practice it is the RF signal that is actually being measured. Also note that the signal on the oscilloscope, called the free-induction decay (FID), is created by the beats of many proton frequencies.

To review briefly the preceding discussion, a tissue at rest has zero net magnetization (*M*). However, in a static external magnetic field, the protons (all magnetic nuclei, in fact) align parallel or antiparallel to the static magnetic field, and because there is a slight magnetization. We can represent this net magnetization as *M*, and because this is aligned along the axis of the static magnetic field, we can indicate

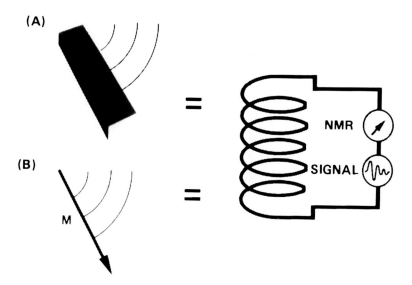

FIG. 3.15. Following the RF pulse, the transverse magnetization M_{xy} precesses around the axis of the external field, inducing an AC signal in the receiver coil in the same way a bar magnet moved in the same plane would induce a signal. Because precession occurs at the Larmor frequency, the voltage induced in the coil is of the same frequency (ω); however, the signal is viewed as beats on the cathode-ray tube (CRT).

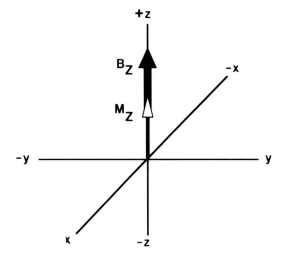

FIG. 3.16. The magnitude and direction of the external magnetic field are represented by a vector (B_z), as are the magnitude and direction of net tissue magnetization (M_z). In this figure, both the external magnetic field and net tissue magnetization are oriented along the z axis, and in many NMR scanners this axis is parallel with the long axis of the body and the long axis of the scanner.

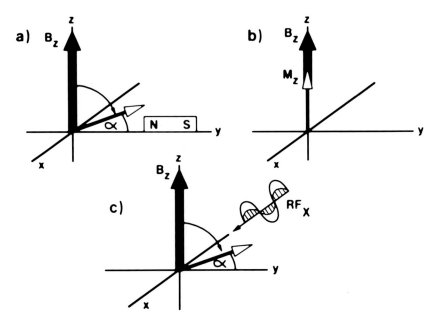

FIG. 3.17. In NMR imaging it is important to be able to change the axis of net tissue magnetization (M_z). One way of approaching this change would be simply to place a bar magnet in the desired direction, in this case, along the y axis (**a**), resulting in a deflection of the net tissue magnetization to a new angle. Moving the bar magnet around in such a fashion would be very difficult within an NMR scanner, and in practice the magnetic force is applied using an electromagnetic wave in the RF range (RF pulse). Recalling from Chapter 2 that the magnetic force acts perpendicular to the line of propagation of the RF wave in order to rotate M_z to the new angle, the pulse should be applied along the x axis, i.e., RF_x.

it as being M_z (Fig. 3.16). One way to change the direction of net magnetization would be simply to apply another magnetic field to the tissue, say with a bar magnet (Fig. 3.17). If applied appropriately along the y axis, this would cause net tissue magnetization to shift slightly from the z axis, with some resultant angle α to the x–y plane.

Another way to accomplish the same result would be to use an RF (electromagnetic) pulse at the resonant frequency of the protons. A proton will precess about the vertical axis of an external magnetic field. If we wish to change the axis for these protons, an RF wave is particularly well suited to applying a constant torque or force. Because the proton is precessing in the main field (often referred to as B_0), the second field needs to oscillate at the precessional frequency in order to apply a constant force. This oscillating magnetic field (often referred to as B_1) is provided by an electromagnetic wave in the RF range, i.e., a radio wave. The magnetic torque, when applied to the proton, causes a rotation about the horizontal axis (Fig. 3.17). The specific resonant frequency is determined by the local value of the magnetic field. During each precessional cycle, the torque due to the radio wave causes the proton axis to rotate slowly (i.e., be deflected) until it eventually lies along the y axis, 90° from where it started. The amount of RF energy needed to do this is called a 90° pulse (Fig. 3.18). The net magnetic moment or magneti-

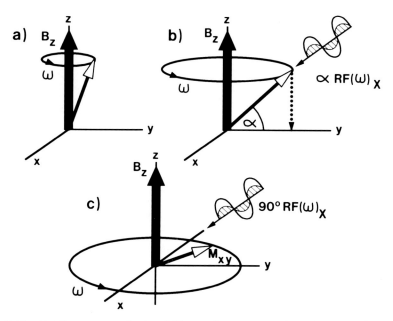

FIG. 3.18. Net tissue magnetization (M_z) actually precesses about the external magnetic field (B_z), and the waveform of the RF pulse is ideal to apply a constant torque to this rotating vector. The amount of rotation is related to the duration and amplitude of the applied RF pulse. An RF pulse of sufficient duration and power to rotate M_z through 90° is referred to as the 90° RF (ω_z) pulse, with ω indicating that the RF pulse needs to be applied at the resonant frequency of the precessing magnetic moment M_z.

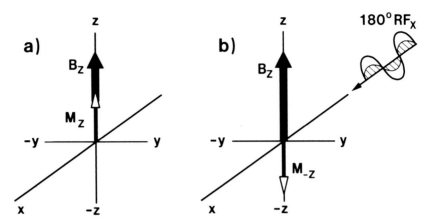

FIG. 3.19. In practical terms, M_z can be rotated through any desired degree of rotation, but commonly the two pulse sequences used are the 180° RF$_x$, resulting in inversion of M_z to M_{-z}, and the 90° RF$_x$.

zation M continues to precess with the same resonant frequency ω in the x–y plane. A precessing magnetic vector induces an NMR signal (Hz) or voltage in a receiver coil if it is precessing perpendicular to the coil, the same way a moving bar magnet produces a voltage in a wire coil (Fig. 3.15). The formula relating these events is $\omega = \gamma B$, where γ is the magnetogyric ratio and B again is the magnetic field. The ω is the resonant angular frequency. It should be remembered that cyclical frequency f is less than the angular frequency: $f = \omega/2\pi$, where ω is the Larmor or characteristic resonant angular frequency.

As might be anticipated, the angle of deflection or rotation of tissue net magnetization (α) depends primarily on the product of the amplitude and length of the applied RF pulse. It is possible to shift the net magnetization vector (M) to any desired angle (α) of deflection by applying the resonant-frequency pulse (α RF) for the appropriate amount of time. The M can, in fact, be completely inverted (Fig. 3.19), and the appropriate pulse is called a 180° RF$_x$ pulse; i.e., 180° RF$_x$ is an RF pulse applied along the x axis to achieve a 180° shift around the x axis.

Images in MRI usually are based on the magnitude of the vector M shown in Fig. 3.18. The type of display shown in Fig. 3.18 can be viewed as polar coordinates. Each point is determined by the vector magnitude M and the angle (α, also called the phase angle) of the vector. An MR image can be produced based on the angle (α,) and these are often useful in measuring flow in blood vessels (see Chapter 6). Images based on M are often called magnitude images, and images based on α are often called imaginary images—the nomenclature can be confusing at times. Imaginary images are useful in displaying the phase angle of the precessing protons. Color can also be used to display phase-angle information on a magnitude image.

When the RF pulse is turned off following a 180° RF pulse, the net tissue magnetization begins to swing back toward the positive z axis, inducing an NMR signal in the appropriately placed receiver coil that must be perpendicular to the moving

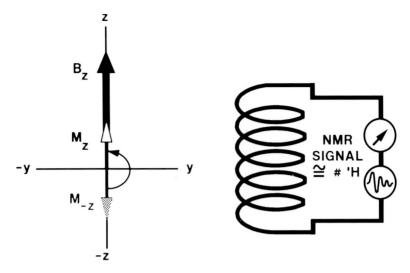

FIG. 3.20. After inversion, M_{-z} returns to M_z after an appropriate time interval. During this process, the magnetic vector changes, and the protons induce the NMR signal (RF signal), which can be detected by a receiver coil, and the signal, viewed as beats rather than the RF frequency, is generally proportional to the number of proton nuclei present in the sample.

magnetic vector (Fig. 3.20). The magnitude of the NMR signal received by the coil is proportional to the number of proton nuclei in the tissue. The time required after the 180° RF$_x$ pulse for the net tissue magnetization to return from negative (M_{-z}) to positive (M_{tz}) is called the *relaxation time* and is referred to in NMR terminology as a relaxation rate T$_1$ or the T$_1$ relaxation time.

T$_1$ Relaxation Time

Proton density, as reviewed earlier, is an important aspect of the NMR signal that conveys much information regarding the chemistry of the substance or tissue being evaluated. The total NMR signal has much more information in it than just the number and type of nuclei reflected in the amplitude of the signal. One can also characterize a given substance or tissue by the way the nuclei relax. Relaxation in NMR refers to the time required for the net tissue magnetization vectors to come to or return to equilibrium conditions in a static external magnetic field.

T$_1$ relaxation can be illustrated by referring back to the compass analogy. A compass needle in the earth's magnetic field will oscillate at a frequency that is characteristic for that needle at a specific point in the earth's magnetic field. At this point we should also consider the duration of oscillation over time. If a compass in the earth's magnetic field has the compass needle subsequently deflected, a damped oscillation of the compass needle is noted. The duration of this decay from beginning to end will have a certain finite time, which we refer to as the relaxation time for the compass needle, or the time required after stimulation for the compass

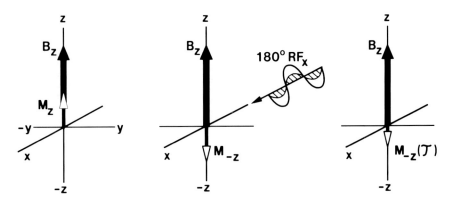

FIG. 3.21. If net tissue magnetization (M_z) is inverted with a 180° RF_x pulse, net tissue magnetization will slowly return from the M_{-z} position to its original M_z position. This process is called relaxation and begins as soon as the 180° RF_z pulse is terminated, as illustrated by the shorter M_{-z} vector that occurs at some time τ after cessation of the 180° RF pulse.

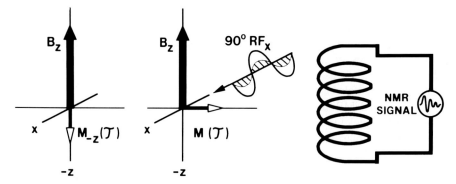

FIG. 3.22. Because of the way most NMR imaging systems are constructed, changes in M_z along the axis cannot be measured directly. Therefore, in this type of imaging, which is referred to as inversion-recovery, a 90° RF_x is applied at variable intervals after the 180° RF_x is applied, so that the signal can be measured from the RF transmitter-receiver coil.

needle to return to equilibrium conditions. Conceptually, T_1 relaxation times in NMR are similar phenomena. For the purposes of illustration, we can return to the vector analysis.

Net tissue magnetization (M_z) is at equilibrium with the external magnetic field B_z. However, if we induce net tissue magnetization to become inverted (M_{-z}) with a bar magnet or, in the case of NMR, with an RF pulse, net tissue magnetization will slowly return to its resting position (M_z). M and any time after M_z inversion to M_{-z} can be represented as either a negative or positive vector along the z axis, and a general case can be illustrated as $M_{-z}a$, with a being some time interval after the initial inversion stimulation (Fig. 3.21).

In practice, changes in net tissue magnetization along the z axis cannot be measured because of the configuration of NMR scanners. Therefore, purely as a prac-

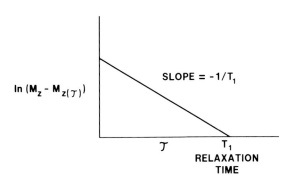

SLOPE = $-1/T_1$

$\ln (M_z - M_{z(\tau)})$

τ T_1

RELAXATION TIME

FIG. 3.23. By obtaining several measurements at variable intervals τ after the 180° RF_x pulse, the time required for M_{-z} to return to M_z can be measured. This time interval is referred to as the T_1 relaxation time, and because it occurs along the z axis, in alignment with the external magnetic field, it is sometimes called the longitudinal relaxation time. The relaxation time is the time constant $1/T_1$. Complete relaxation occurs at approximately $3T_1$ to $4T_1$.

tical technique in measuring T_1, M_z is deflected toward the coil by following the 180° RF pulse with a 90° pulse (Fig. 3.22). This process is repeated for several different time intervals (t) following the initial M_z inversion, and the magnitude of M_{-z} is measured with each repetition. After several measurements, T_1 can be determined, as illustrated in Fig. 3.23. Because this relaxation occurs along the $_z$ axis or is parallel to or longitudinal with the static magnetic field, this form of T_1 relaxation is sometimes referred to as *longitudinal relaxation.* It is also called spin-lattice relaxation time, because during the relaxation process, energy in the form of heat is lost through molecular collisions to the surrounding tissue (lattice). Thus, we have now two NMR methods to describe a given tissue or sample. One is the density of the nuclei (proton nuclei within that sample), and the second is the time it takes the net magnetization of the tissue or sample to return to its equilibrium position along the z axis after some magnetic deflection.

T_2 Relaxation Time

The third parameter is T_2. Everyone has had the experience of throwing a pebble in a small pond and watching the wave spread out in a circular fashion until it has traversed the entire surface of the pond. The time is dependent on the size of the pond, and if the pond is not too large, the wave is visible throughout its course over the surface. If we take a handful of pebbles, however, and throw them into the pond, the effect of the waveforms on the surface is quite different. Although each wave initially starts out as did the single wave from the single pebble, the wave fronts very quickly encounter each other, leaving no discernible single wave, and the surface again "appears" smoother. In fact, this is not true; the waves are still traversing the surface, but because of superimposition, the crests and troughs tend to cancel each other out. This wave interference is similar to the proton-vector cancellation that occurs in T_2 relaxation.

Waveform interference can also be illustrated by tuning forks. If, for example, we took a room full of tuning forks all tuned to the tone C and struck each one of

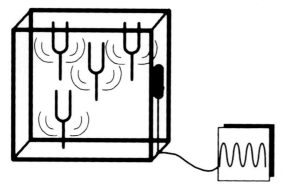

FIG. 3.24. Tuning forks tuned to the same tone enclosed in a room, if struck, will emit a loud tone that can be detected by a microphone.

FIG. 3.25. If tuning forks that originally were tuned to the same tone have variable small weights attached to their arms, and then are induced to vibrate, a microphone enclosed within the room will detect no tone at all because of the phase interference among the tuning forks produced by the small weights. If one of the tuning forks is removed from the room, however, a tone will be recorded, because the dampening effect of wave interference will have been removed. In NMR scanning, T_2 relaxation involves a similar kind of cancellation among proton magnetic moments that rapidly dephase.

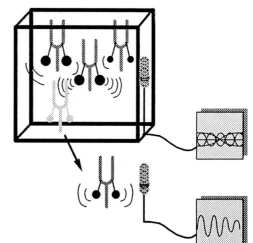

them individually and simultaneously, we should have a very loud C tone, with loudness proportional to the number of tuning forks in the room (Fig. 3.24). If, instead, we took a soldering iron and applied various amounts of solder to all of the tuning forks, so that each resonant tone was just slightly different than the tone C, and again struck all of the tuning forks simultaneously, we should initially hear a loud mixed tone. The sound waves would not reinforce each other, however, and we should hear a confusing waxing and waning muted sound. If we removed one of the tuning forks from the room, we again would hear the constant single tone: the tone emanating from the single tuning fork (Fig. 3.25).

This sonic interference is similar to the disruption in the visual pattern of the waves on the surface of the pond. Because each of the tuning forks was tuned slightly differently because of the applied solder, the sonic waves did not reinforce each other, but rather dephased very quickly. In NMR, the explanation of T_2 relaxation time also involves dephasing phenomena, although it is the precessional frequencies of the protons in the transverse plane that are dephasing in the NMR example. Following a 90° RF pulse, the protons precess together in the x–y plane and produce a "loud" signal. The signal intensity (loudness) decreases quickly because of dephasing of the protons, just as the solder on the tuning-fork arms produced dephasing of the tone. As a result of proton dephasing, the net magnetization vector in the transverse plane decreases to zero very quickly because of the cancellation of net magnetization. T_2 relaxation time is thus a time-constant measurement of the cancellation of the individual magnetic moments of the precessing protons, rather than a waveform interference.

In MRI, before application of the static external magnetic field, the magnetic moments of the nuclei making up the tissue are randomly aligned, as previously discussed. When a magnetic field is applied, individual protons align with the direction of the applied magnetic field B_z, but precess around it. As these magnetic moments are randomly distributed around the z axis, the proton vectors in the xy plane cancel one another out, and $M_{xy} = 0$, while the M_z components along the direction of the applied magnetic field do not cancel each other and produce a net magnetic moment M_z (Fig. 3.26). If an RF pulse at the resonant frequency of the precessing nuclei is broadcast into the tissue, two things occur simultaneously:

1. The net tissue magnetization (M_z) will be rotated away from the z axis, as shown in Fig. 3.27. The angle of rotation, α, depends primarily on the duration and power of the applied RF pulse ($\alpha = Kt_p$, where t_p is the pulse length, in seconds, and K is a constant).
2. The individual magnetic moments are brought into the same phase (coherence) with each other, and the net magnetic moment (M) then precesses at the resonant frequency in the x–y plane.

If this sample is within the RF receiver coil and M_{xy} is precessing perpendicular to it, an NMR signal will be recorded. The amplitude of the initial signal A_0 will depend on the magnitude of the component of M (M_{xy} in the x–y plane). The amplitude (A) of this signal decays in an exponential natural log (e) fashion with time, t ($A = A_0 e^{-t/T_2}$), as the individual magnetic moments dephase or lose coherence. T_2 relaxation time is the characteristic or average decay time for the process.

Following a 90° RF pulse, the mean vector M is seen to lie along the y axis (Fig. 3.27). When the RF field is turned off, the proton magnetic moments start to realign with the large external magnetic field B. At any time during realignment, the magnetization M can be considered to be a vector composed of a transverse component M_{xy} and a longitudinal component M_z. Following the 90° RF pulse, the transverse component of magnetization M_z decays quickly to zero as the longitudinal component M_z slowly grows to its original value. The rate of decay of the transverse magnetization M_{xy} is exponential, with the time constant T_2, the transverse relaxation time (Fig. 3.28). The rate of growth of M_z along the longitudinal axis is also exponential, with the time constant T_1, the longitudinal relaxation time.

T_2 is a measure of how long the substance maintains the temporary transverse magnetization, which is perpendicular to the external magnetic field. Magnetic inhomogeneity causes T_2 relaxation. T_2 indicates the relationship between the strength and inhomogeneity of the tissue magnetic field and the amount of resonance inter-

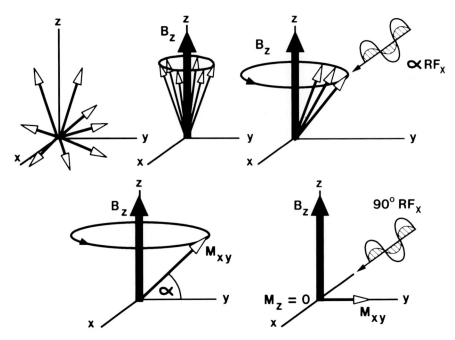

FIG. 3.26. The magnetic moments of the randomly aligned protons precess about the z axis in the presence of an external magnetic field (B_z). This orientation results in a net tissue magnetization along the z axis (M_z), but because they are randomly aligned with respect to the x–y axes, no magnetic moment is recorded in the x–y plane. However, when an RF pulse is applied, two things occur simultaneously. First, the net tissue magnetization begins to rotate about the x axis; second, the RF pulse causes the randomly aligned proton magnetic moments to become coherent with respect to the x–y plane, and they tend to precess together. If the RF pulse applied is appropriate for a 90° rotation (90° RF_x), then the magnetic moments will be coherently aligned on the x–y plane, resulting in a magnetic moment in the x–y plane (M_{xy}), but no net tissue magnetization will be recorded on the z axis ($M_z = 0$). Note: In the static reference frame, M_z spirals down to the x–y plane.

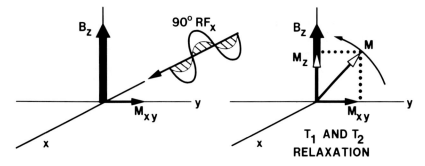

FIG. 3.27. After the 90° RF pulse is terminated, tissue magnetization begins to relax (both the M_{xy} and M_z) and, at any time after the RF_x pulse, can be thought of as having vector components of M_z and M_{xy}. M_{xy} is lost or relaxes by virtue of the individual proton magnetic moments precessing about the z axis at different rates and therefore losing phase coherence (T_2 relaxation), whereas M_z relaxation occurs by a realignment of M along the z axis (T_1 relaxation). Note: In the static frame of reference, M actually spirals upward around the z axis until full relaxation, when it again precesses around z.

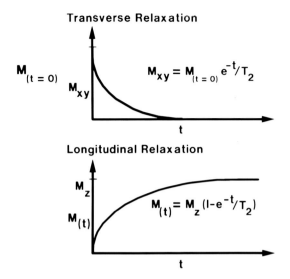

Transverse Relaxation

$$M_{xy} = M_{(t=0)} e^{-t/T_2}$$

$M_{(t=0)}$

M_{xy}

t

Longitudinal Relaxation

$$M_{(t)} = M_z (1 - e^{-t/T_2})$$

M_z

$M_{(t)}$

t

FIG. 3.28. T_2 relaxation is a decay of net magnetization in the M_{xy} plane, with an exponential time constant T_2 or transverse relaxation time, wheras longitudinal relaxation along the z axis is a rate of growth of M along the z axis, with time constant T_1, or the longitudinal relaxation time.

action occurring between precessing protons in the tissue. Protons maintaining the transverse magnetization are coherent, or rotating in phase about the vertical axis. Phase coherence of the protons is destroyed by inhomogeneous external magnetic fields, resonance flipping of protons precessing at the same frequency, and local internal magnetic fields.

Following a 90° RF_x pulse, the signal (FID, see next section) vanishes because the transverse component of the magnetization decays. If the magnetic fields were really homogeneous, the decay constant would be equal to T_2, the transverse relaxation time. This situation is unrealistic, and in practice the magnetic fields generated by magnets have some inhomogeneity. The effective time constant governing signal decay, T_2^*, is therefore always shorter than T_2.

The second process affecting the time evolution of the dephasing of transverse magnetization results from the interactions among the nuclei themselves. Nuclei produce small incremental magnetic fields that also cause dephasing of M_{xy}. This is an intrinsic process; that is, it is independent of instrumental imperfections. It is a random process, governed solely by the random flipping of two neighboring protons that are precessing at the same frequency, or, in other words, spin-spin relaxation time T_2. The importance of T_2^* and T_2 in MRI is that T_2^*, the incoherence due to external-field inhomogeneity, is reversible, but T_2 is not reversible.

Free-Induction Decay

One of the most fundamental examples of a pulsed NMR experiment is illustrated by free-induction decay (FID). An RF pulse at the resonant frequency rotates the M_z vector out of the z direction, and when the pulse is terminated, one observes an oscillating sine-wave signal [$\sin(\omega t)$] that decreases in amplitude in exponential fashion with time (e^{-t/T_2}), as shown in Fig. 3.29. Essentially, in this example, the

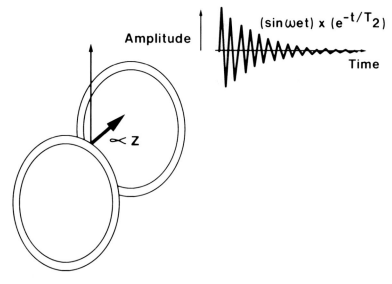

FIG. 3.29. Following a 90° RF pulse, the fundamental NMR signal recorded is a damped-amplitude wave that decays with time constant T_2 and is referred to as FID and as such represents one of the most fundamental experiments in NMR spectroscopy.

amplitude of the signal that corresponds to the number of protons in the tissue is recorded as an oscillating sine-wave voltage (beats), and the signal is recorded over the period during which that signal is induced. Thus, this is an amplitude-versus-time plot and is referred to as the FID signal. The FID decays exponentially in a homogeneous external magnetic field. Because the external field is not homogeneous, however, it is to be noted that while the FID signal decays with a time constant T_2^*, the echo amplitude decays with a time constant T_2, the true spin-spin relaxation time.

To state this important principle in a slightly different way, in NMR it is the transverse magnetization, M_{xy} (according to Faraday's law of induction), that can induce a voltage in a receiver coil. By contrast, the longitudinal magnetization is static and thus does not meet the requirements for magnetic induction. Keeping protons in the longitudinal position can be important to eliminate tissue signals such as the static tissue suppression desired in imaging blood flow in vessels. Once the 90° RF_x pulse is removed, the magnetization is subjected to the effect of the static magnetic field (B) only, and thus precesses about it. During this postexcitation or free-precession period, after the RF field has been turned off, the magnetic moment can induce voltage in a receiver coil, situated in the transverse plane. Because precession occurs at the Larmor frequency, the voltage induced in the coil circuit is of the same frequency. However, the transverse magnetization M_{xy} does not persist. It decays to zero, with a characteristic time constant (T_2), and so does the amplitude of the detected voltage (Fig. 3.29). For this reason, the signal is called FID, manifesting itself as a damped signal oscillation or beats. Because the initial signal amplitude is proportional to the transverse magnetization, which is itself proportional to the number of nuclei excited in a particular voxel of tissue, differences in hydrogen density become discernible in the NMR image.

Inversion-Recovery Technique

An extension of this discussion suggests that most NMR experiments divide naturally into two periods: periods of excitation and periods of induction or "listening" in which the RF signal from the sample is observed (Fig. 3.30). If this delay time is made too short, however, there is a decrease in initial amplitude, A_0, observed in the subsequent experiment. This happens because insufficient time is allowed for longitudinal relaxation, and M_z is not fully recovered to the equilibrium value. This provides a useful technique for evaluating T_1 with a preparative excitation technique.

Measurement of T_1. As noted earlier, by adjusting the length of the RF pulse, we achieve a 90° RF_x that gives the maximum possible signal amplitude, A_0, in the xy plane (M_{xy}). By doubling the length ($2 \times 90° RF_x$), we can rotate M through 180°, or, in fact, any angle α desired (αRF_x). The magnitude of the longitudinal net magnetization M_z then varies as a function of time in an exponential fashion, with the rate constant $1/T_1$.

As noted previously, because of the way NMR scanners are configured, longitudinal relaxation along the z axis cannot be observed directly. Only vectors moving perpendicular to the RF coil will generate an NMR signal. Thus, in practice, to observe the relaxation along the z axis, a second 90° RF pulse must be applied to the sample during recovery (Fig. 3.30). One can measure the actual time required

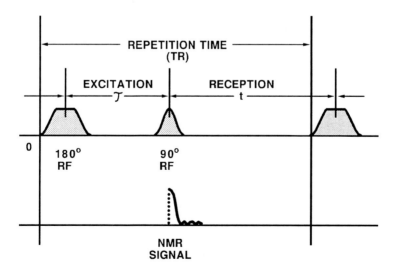

FIG. 3.30. Many imaging schemes are used in MRI. However, these experiments naturally divide into two periods: a period of excitation or irradiation of the tissue with RF pulses and a period during which the RF coils are tuned to listen for the NMR signal. The period of time between the sets of tissue irradiation is referred to as the repetition time (T_{rep} or TR).

for longitudinal relaxation along the z axis by following the 180° pulse with variably spaced 90° pulses. This method is called *inversion recovery* (i.e., inversion of the magnetization from M_z to M_{-z}, and then subsequent recovery or relaxation). In practice, multiple averages are taken for each 180°-to-90° interval. However, the time between pulse pairs, or the repetition rate, is kept long to allow total recovery of the tissue between RF excitations. This method is more sensitive to differences in T_1 than is saturation recovery (a series of 90° RF_x pulses, see Appendix I).

The inversion-recovery technique is used in some MRI experiments to give an evaluation of T_1 or to increase the T_1 weighting of the image. In addition, there are other preparative excitation sequences using alternative pulsing arrangements to deliver other types of NMR data, as we shall see in the section on imaging.

Spin-Echo Technique

Many explanations of the spin-echo technique use a rotating frame of reference, which rotates with the precessing nuclear moments, to study the relative magnetic-vector changes. In some cases this makes the motion of the net magnetization easier to understand, but in some respects it is confusing, and in this section T_2 will be discussed using a static frame of reference. However, those readers going on to other texts should be sure to determine if the author is discussing the spin-echo technique using a rotating frame or a static frame of reference.

We have discussed the tendency of a top in a gravitational field to wobble or precess around the gravitational field. Similarly, ensembles of protons with magnetic moments tend to align with and precess around an externally applied static magnetic field. As opposed to FID, the spin-echo is an RF signal that returns (echoes) after a delay. The amplitude of the spin-echo is directly related to the number of protons in the tissue irradiated and how well they remain in phase. The form of the echo display is a mirror image of the FID.

The spin-echo is produced by first exposing a tissue that has been placed in a static external magnetic field to a 90° RF pulse along the x axis (90° RF_x). The magnetization M of the excited volume that was pointing along the z axis is now rotated 90° so that it points along the y axis. After the 90° RF_x pulse, M precesses about the z axis at the same precessional frequency (ω). Small variations in the external magnetic field in the excited tissue cause some protons to experience slightly stronger and some slightly weaker magnetic fields. Those in the stronger local magnetic fields, M_H, are going to precess at a slightly higher frequency than those in the weaker local magnetic field, M_T. As the protons lose coherence or phase, those in the weaker field (M_T) will move more slowly and lag behind those experiencing a slightly higher field (M_H). After an interval (τ) following the 90° RF_x, the sample is exposed to a 180° pulse from the RF_x coil that causes a further 180° rotation about the x axis. This results in the y component of the magnetization vector changing sign, while the x component is unaffected. Following this 180° RF_x, vectors M_H and M_T continue to precess in the counterclockwise direction. However, the effect of the 180° pulse is such that the slower-precessing vectors are in front of the faster-precessing vectors, and the faster overtake the slower with a crescendo–decrescendo echo recorded as the spin-echo, with the vectors coming into and then losing coherence. This signal height is proportional to the proton density and T_2 and is called the *spin-echo*.

We can appreciate this relationship somewhat better if we shift our conventional frame of reference and take a position high on the z axis and look down at the x–y plane. The faster-moving vectors can be represented by those attached to the hare (M_H), and the slower by those attached to the tortoise (M_T). The longer the two are allowed to "race," the farther ahead the hare will be. If we were to pick up the vector of the tortoise and the hare, such that their relative positions along the y axis were the same, but the tortoise was ahead of the hare at some point, the hare would catch up with the tortoise, and the two vectors would be coherent again for a short period of time. At that point the amplitude along the y axis would be the greatest, and a signal would be recorded. Because the progress of the faster-moving hare causes him to overtake and then pass the tortoise, there is an ascending signal to maximum coherence, and a descending signal, giving a mirror image of an FID configuration (Fig. 3.31). In MRI, this effect of changing the positions of the tortoise and the hare is achieved by a 180° RF_x pulse. This can be repeated as many times as necessary for adequate imaging or measurement of T_2.

In summary, the spin-echo is produced by a 90° RF pulse followed by a 180° RF pulse. The FID resulting from saturation-recovery or inversion-recovery sequences can also be converted to a spin-echo if a 180° pulse follows the last 90° pulse. The strength of the spin-echo depends on hydrogen density and T_2. T_1 information weighting in images can be adjusted by variation of the time between pulse pairs (i.e., TR, the repetition rate).

Measurement of T_2. Measurement of T_2 using the spin-echo technique was first proposed by Hahn in 1950 in *Physics Review*, using the 90°, τ, 180° sequence, and subsequent observation at a time TE (2τ) of an "echo." After the 90° RF_x pulse, the precessional frequencies are in phase, but very quickly begin to fan out as some of the nuclei precess faster than others. At a time τ after the 90° pulse, a 180° pulse is applied, as we have seen in the spin-echo sequence, which has the effect of placing the more rapidly precessing magnetic moments behind the slower. At a time 2τ, all the individual magnetic moments come into phase, and the continuing movement causes them again to lose phase coherence. The reshaping of the fanned-out magnetic moments (M) causes a free-induction signal to build to a maximum at 2τ. If transverse relaxation did not occur, the echo amplitude might be just as large as the initial value of the free induction following the 90° pulse, but some magnetic-moment (M) coherence decreases during the time 2τ because of the natural process responsible for transverse relaxation in the time T_2. Thus, the echo amplitude depends on T_2, and for a sample with only a single resonant frequency, T_2 may in principle be determined from a plot of a series of peak echo amplitudes. In the more general case, however, because the echo is just two FIDs back-to-back, Fourier transformation of half the echo results in a spectrum with line heights dependent on their individual T_2 values. As in the measurement of T_1 by the 180° $RF_x \times \tau \times$ 90° RF_x method, it is necessary to carry out a separate pulse sequence for each

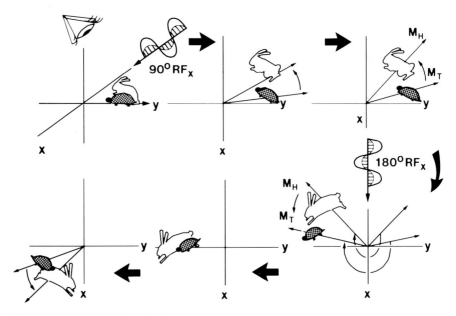

FIG. 3.31. The NMR signal in the spin-echo technique is produced because of the fact that following the 90° RF$_x$ pulse, all proton magnetic moments are in phase in the x–y plane, but subsequently, because of local variations in the magnetic field, some of the protons precess faster (M_H) than others (M_T). However, if a subsequent 180° RF$_x$ pulse is broadcast into the sample, the individual magnetic moments undergo a 180° rotation about or around the x axis, which results in the faster-precessing magnetic moments being behind the slower ones. A crescendo–decrescendo (echo) signal is produced as these faster magnetic moments over-take, stay briefly in phase with, and then pass beyond the slower magnetic moments. The time required for this phase coherence to be reestablished is exactly equal to the elapsed time between the 90° RF$_x$ and the 180° RF$_x$ pulses. This tissue irradiation can be repeated several times; however, coherence of the NMR signal in the spin-echo technique is lost be-cause of two processes: (1) Because of inhomogeneities in the fluctuating internal field of the substance produced by magnetic dipoles in the nuclei and resonance spin-spin flipping, and this loss cannot be reconstituted. Therefore, over time, the NMR spin-echo signal de-creases in intensity. (2) Because of inhomogeneities in the external magnetic field. Because the phase incoherence induced by the external magnetic field is constant, it can be recon-stituted. To summarize, transverse magnetization is lost by two processes: rapidly because of nonuniformity in the external magnetic field produced by the NMR scanner (designated $T_2{}^*$ and more slowly because of internal-field nonuniformity due to characteristics of the tis-sue (designated $T_2{}^*$). Inhomogeneity in the external field (T_2) determines the width of the spin-echo, and T_2 determines the height of successive echoes.

value of τ and wait between pulse sequences to allow adequate time (at least 5 $\times$ T_1) for restoration of equilibrium.

The spin-echo technique is influenced in its range of applicability because of the effect of molecular diffusion. The precise refocussing of all precessing magnetic moments (M) is dependent on each nucleus remaining in a constant magnetic field during the time of the experiment. If diffusion causes nuclei to move from one part of an inhomogeneous field to another, the echo amplitude is reduced. Diffusion coefficients are thus readily measured by spin-echo technique. The Carr-Purcell method for measuring T_2 is an improvement on the simple spin-echo technique. This method uses 180° pulses that are applied at τ, 2τ, 3τ, 5τ, etc., to form echoes at 2τ, 4τ, 6τ, etc. The height of the echoes may be measured in short time intervals to preclude appreciable diffusion. Actually, small missettings of pulses will cause cumulative errors that can be overcome by a shift in RF phase, which is the Meiboom-Gill method.

Spatial Encoding

The NMR principles discussed thus far are used in NMR spectroscopy, but the output is still in the form of spectroscopic lines. The question is how to process the data to obtain a medical image. The problem at this point is to find some way to locate in space the source of the NMR signal. If that were possible, then within the scanning area we could assign a given signal back to a certain location and from there reconstruct a cross-sectional image, as in the CT analogy. What is needed is some sort of spatial encoding of the NMR signal. It is probably easiest to understand how this is done if we again borrow a bit more from the tuning-fork analogy. If a C tuning fork is placed in a room in which there are several tuning forks that have different tones (resonant frequencies), for example, the notes F, A, C, and E, indicated in Fig. 3.32, and again strike the C tuning fork, a peculiar phenomenon occurs. Even though they are all tuning forks, only the tuning fork that emits the letter C will begin to vibrate (resonate). All of the other tuning forks seem to ignore the presence of the vibrating C tuning fork in the room.

It will be recalled from the section on electromagnetic waves that frequency and energy are directly related. What is occurring in this tuning-fork example is that energy is imparted to the C tuning fork as we strike it with the mallet. This energy is then transformed into sonic waves with a certain frequency (cycles per second or hertz), which we hear as the tone or the note C, and the note's amplitude is heard

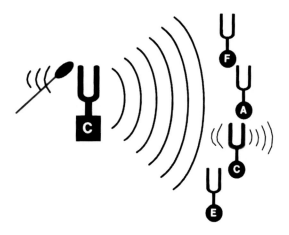

FIG. 3.32. If several tuning forks are placed in proximity to a tuning fork that has been struck with a mallet, only the tuning fork with the same tone (resonant frequency) will absorb the specific or characteristic energy and begin to resonate. The other tuning forks are not capable of absorbing the energy from an unmatched tone. In other words, the energy exchange must occur at a very specific or characteristic frequency or tone.

as the loudness of the note C. This energy is then transmitted across the room to all the tuning forks present, but only the C tuning fork is able to absorb that specific energy, and that energy causes the arms to vibrate, subsequently reemitting (resonating) the appropriate frequency, the tone C. Throughout this book, many of the principles of magnetic resonance will be explained in terms of analogies with sound waves. It is important to remember, however, that sonic waves are not electromagnetic waves. But they do have certain characteristics analogous to electromagnetic waves: wavelength, frequency, and amplitude.

Carrying these concepts further and extending them to the NMR sample or *in vitro* tissue experiments, the protons or nuclei generally are in an unaligned state, with zero magnetization. However, when a tissue is placed in an external static magnetic field, the protons align with the external magnetic field. If, as in Fig. 3.33, some are receptive and able to resonate when a signal of a specific frequency is applied to the tissue, in this case, "hello," they will be excited to a higher energy

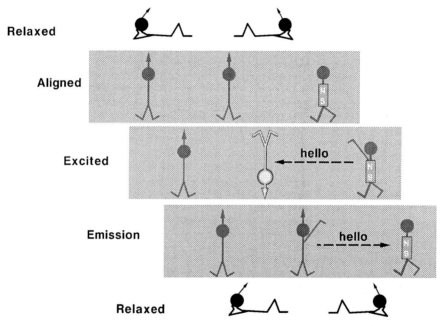

FIG. 3.33. Protons, in the absence of an external magnetic field, are randomly aligned, with no net tissue magnetization; however, when placed in the presence of an external magnetic field, they become aligned with the field and can be induced (excited) to change alignment by absorption of a signal of specific frequency, in this case, "hello." The protons, after some period of time, then lose the energy and become realigned in their initial orientation. During this process, an antenna can record an emitted signal from the protons that has the same signal frequency ("hello"). The frequency signal is actually present within the spinning protons, and the input perturbation induces the emitted signal ("hello" in the illustration). Removal of the external magnetic field will again lead to random alignment of the protons and zero net magnetization. In remembering MRI principles using this analogy, it is important to note that in MRI the RF excitation signal induces the protons to tilt into a position such that the receiver can detect the signal. The signal, however, is a function of the number and precessional frequency of the protons already present within the tissue.

state antiparallel to the static magnetic field. Some time later, however, they will flip back to the parallel lower energy level, and in the process a signal of the same frequency can be detected by an antenna. Removal of the magnetic field will again allow a random alignment of the protons in the tissue and zero net magnetization.

Magnetic resonance, however, implies an interaction between magnetic fields, rather than a physical interaction of sonic waves. For most of us, the most familiar interaction of a magnet with a magnetic field is the interaction of a compass needle (permanent bar magnet mounted on a needle fulcrum) with the magnetic field of the earth. At rest, the compass needle is aligned with the earth's magnetic field, pointing north. If the compass needle is deflected with a finger, it will swing back toward its resting position, overshoot, and oscillate back and forth at some frequency, eventually coming to rest, again pointing north. This frequency of oscillation is called the natural frequency, and for any given point in the magnetic field of any given compass needle, the frequency is characteristic. Because of this relationship between a compass needle's natural frequency and the magnetic field of the earth, we can determine with this system our latitude on the earth or spatial location. If our compass had a natural frequency of 1 Hz at the equator, with 0.3 G field strength, and if we moved to a new position in which the natural frequency was 2 Hz, we would know we were at a latitude that was near the north pole corresponding to a magnetic field strength twice that at the equator, or 0.6 G magnetic field strength. We would also know whether we were north or south of the equator by determining whether we were traveling toward or away from the north-pointing compass in getting to the new position (Fig. 3.34). In other words, using the frequency of the compass, we can determine (spatially encode) our latitudinal position. In NMR imaging, the magnet is, of course, not a compass needle, but rather the magnetic moment of an atomic nucleus, usually hydrogen. The magnetic field in NMR is a very strong magnetic field, approximately 4,000 to 40,000 times that of the earth or greater, induced by the surrounding magnet of the NMR imaging system.

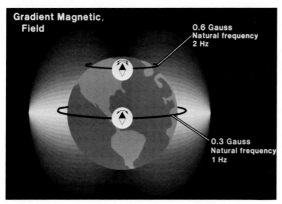

FIG. 3.34. A compass needle at the equator experiencing a magnetic field of approximately 0.3 G will oscillate at its natural frequency after it is deflected. This natural frequency of oscillation is influenced by the magnetic field in which the compass is placed, such that doubling the magnetic field will double the natural frequency of oscillation. In this way, if we were given a natural frequency of 1 Hz at the equator and placed in a new position on the earth in which the natural frequency of oscillation was observed to have increased to 2 Hz, we could correctly locate our position at that latitude corresponding to exactly twice the magnetic field of the equator, or 0.6 G.

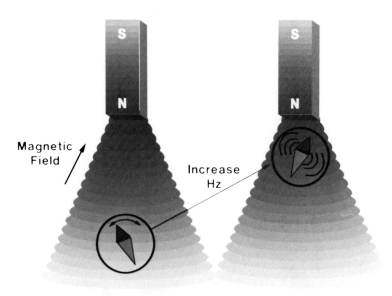

FIG. 3.35. The strength of the magnetic field will influence the natural (resonant) frequency of vibration of a compass needle such that if the compass is moved closer to the magnet and into a higher field strength, the frequency will increase. This predictable relationship between frequency and magnetic field strength is the mechanism by which NMR information is spatially encoded. In other words, the frequency has spatially encoded information.

The potential for spatial encoding of a magnetic field is similarly demonstrated when a deflected compass needle is noted to oscillate at its resonant (natural) frequency in the magnetic field of a bar magnet (Fig. 3.35). When the compass needle is advanced toward the magnet, the resonant frequency increases. The result is that the frequency of oscillation (new resonant frequency) increases, and it is the increasing strength of the magnetic field of the bar magnet that has produced the change. The gradient coils in the imaging system produce these required variations in magnetic field strength, and the protons, rather than compass needle, respond with proportional changes in precessional frequency.

The principle of NMR incorporates the concept of exciting tissue with RF electromagnetic waves and "listening" with an antenna or RF coil for the resonant frequency of the nuclear species excited. To illustrate how the RF signal is processed, let us assume for the moment that we have an imaginary tissue that is composed of small TV receiver-transmitters instead of protons. The TV station WNMR broadcasts the programs "60 Minutes," "News," and "Sports" with the same radio frequency and beams the channel at the TV receiver-transmitters within the tissue. Each TV-set receiver-transmitter will pick up the programs and visually transmit all three programs to an off-site viewer. We, the viewers, will know that we have three channel selections, A, B, and C, but because we are receiving all three programs on each channel, we have no idea where the receiving antenna is within the tissue (Fig. 3.36).

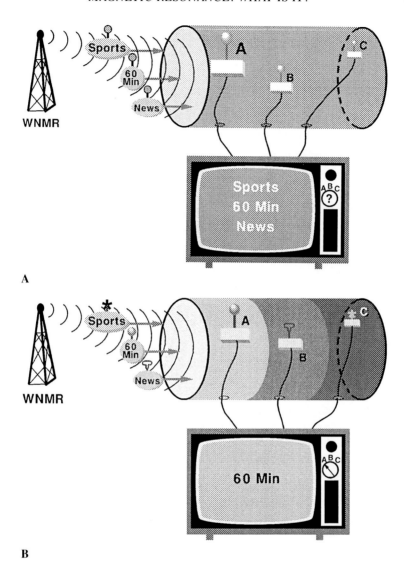

A

B

FIG. 3.36. In NMR, each proton within the tissue acts as a small transmitter that is induced by an RF signal to transmit a characteristic signal. If a TV station WNMR is broadcasting three programs ("News," "60 Minutes," and "Sports") on the same frequency, we are unable to determine the position of a receiver-transmitter antenna within a sample or tissue by turning the TV dial to the three receiver-transmitters to which we are connected. However, if each receiver-transmitter is equipped with a similarly matched antenna, then, when the dial is turned, only the A channel will receive "60 Minutes," and we can identify the spatial position of that receiver-transmitter. In MRI, the selectivity of the antenna of the protons is established by applying a gradient magnetic field. The RF pulse in MRI actually tilts the protons so that the receiver can detect the signal frequency prescribed by the gradient coils.

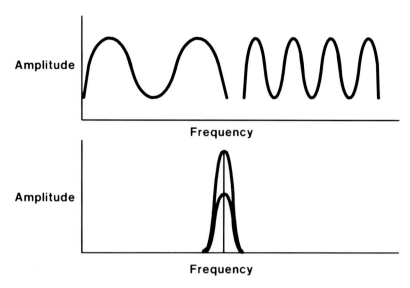

FIG. 3.37. In NMR imaging, RF waves in the NMR signal can have the same amplitude but different frequencies (**top**), or two waves can have the same frequency but different amplitudes, and they can potentially be distinguished from each other on this basis.

However, if WNMR changes its programming policy and assigns a signal of different frequency for each program and we equip each receiving station with the appropriate UHF, VHF, or short-wave antenna, only receiver A will receive "60 Minutes," only receiver B will pick up "News," and only receiver C will receive "Sports." Now, by turning the dial on our channel selector, we know when we get "60 Minutes" that it corresponds to receiver-transmitter A, and similarly we have some idea where within the tissue the receiver-transmitters are located.

In NMR imaging, the principles are not very different from those described in the TV analogy. We are able to determine where a given proton is located in space by a technique that is similar to changing the antenna to fit a certain TV channel (resonant frequency), and the method that allows us to perform this is to superimpose a magnetic gradient on the static magnetic field. As reviewed earlier, the frequency of magnetic resonance for a specific nuclear species is dependent on the strength of the magnetic field ($\omega = \gamma B$). This is specifically given by the Larmor equation, where the field-frequency relation for hydrogen is 42.58 MHz/T. All forms of NMR imaging use some type of spatially encoded frequency discrimination to allow formation of the image. The major concept to bear in mind is that the stronger the magnetic field, the higher the precessional resonant frequency, and thus the higher the energy exchanged when flipping between low and high energy states.

In NMR imaging, electromagnetic waves can exist as single monochromatic frequencies, and two waves with the same amplitude can be discriminated from each other if they have different frequencies (Fig. 3.37). The same wave can be represented in one of two ways: either as a wave of given amplitude and duration (time

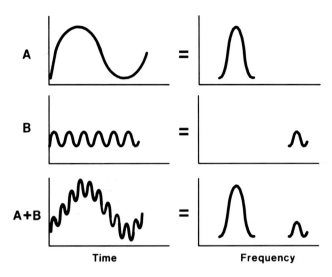

Time   **Frequency**

FIG. 3.38. RF electromagnetic waves in the NMR signal usually are modulated or super-imposed on each other, resulting in complex amplitudes and frequencies, as illustrated in the time domain of A + B. Fortunately, using a complex mathematical digital-computer pro-gram called the fast Fourier transform, these complex-amplitude waveforms in the time do-main can be converted to separable-amplitude waveforms in the frequency domain, and this frequency resolution can be used to locate the part of the body from which the RF signal was sent.

domain) or as a frequency distribution of waves (frequency domain) (Fig. 3.38). In addition, many waves of different frequencies and amplitudes can be superimposed on each other and represented as one wave with frequency and amplitude modula-tion. In NMR imaging, these characteristics of frequency and amplitude or energy are used to make images of the body by separating a complex series of RF signals emitted from the nuclei into their components of frequency and amplitude. The frequency is used to locate a particular position of the nucleus within the body, and the amplitude is used to determine the number of nuclei present at that location.

Representation of the FID curve by its component frequencies amounts to trans-forming the amplitude-versus-time information of the FID into a plot of amplitude versus frequency. This is usually accomplished by using a Fourier transform, named for the French mathematician Jean Baptiste Fourier (digital Fourier transform, DFT) (Fig. 3.39). In the frequency domain in NMR spectroscopy, a narrow spectral line with a narrow peak and long tail is referred to as a *Lorentzian line*. In actual appli-cation, all of the frequencies coming from an excited sample or tissue are measured simultaneously, and the information is sent to a computer that analyzes the signal strength at each of the frequencies of interest.

In NMR, the use of a linear-gradient magnetic field sets up a certain relationship between frequency and position. The concept of utilizing a linear gradient in the magnetic field in conjunction with an image-reconstruction technique, which had

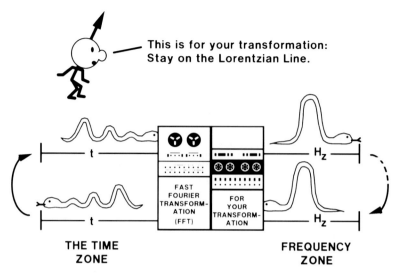

FIG. 3.39. In NMR image reconstruction it is important to change the radio-wave NMR signal from an amplitude–time display (time zone) to an amplitude–frequency display (frequency domain), because the frequency is used to locate the signal in space, whereas the amplitude is used to determine the number of protons present in that space. This transformation is performed using a sophisticated computer algorithm called the Fourier transformation (FT). Using the FT is analogous to separating white light onto its color components with a prism.

previously been used in conjunction with CT scanning, i.e., filtered back-projection, was put forward by Lauterbur in a 1973 article in *Nature*. To reconstruct a three-dimensional image of the body, three such linear gradients are used that are perpendicular to each other. Nevertheless, the general principle, as we have just reviewed, is to relate a specific frequency to a specific geometric location. The difference between the NMR imaging process and the spectroscopic process is that in NMR imaging, each point is located with a specific frequency by gradient coil.

We shall discuss filtered back-projection and other reconstruction imaging techniques in more detail in the next chapter. However, the method is somewhat analogous to the problem of trying to determine the configuration of an object placed inside a lamp shade and tracing its contours on the shade in several different places and subsequently projecting back to the intersection of all of these traced images to define the location and configuration of the object itself. In general, the more tracings that are made to try to define the configuration (the more angles of view or the more projections), the more accurate the final configuration is likely to be. The amplitude of radio waves used in NMR, as opposed to the light waves used in the lamp-shade problem, corresponds to the amount of material (hydrogen) at a given location. In other words, the frequency indicates the spatial location, and the amplitude indicates the amount of material present.

We can represent the spatial encoding in NMR as in Fig. 3.40. The object is placed in a static magnetic field (*B*), and subsequently a gradient magnetic field is

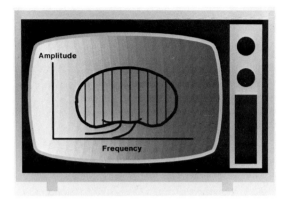

FIG. 3.40. In NMR imaging, the RF signal has amplitude information that corresponds to the number of hydrogen nuclei present. The frequency of the RF signal can be used to locate the nuclei in space because of the fact that the frequency increases with increasing magnetic field strength. Thus, the signal, in this case from a conceptualized kidney, can be thought of as an amplitude–frequency plot from which the general outline and character of the tissue can be determined.

applied. Planes in the figure correspond to higher or lower positions on the gradient magnetic field. This results in correspondingly higher or lower resonant frequencies, respectively, and these frequencies can be related back to the gradient magnetic field, and the corresponding spatial locations of the planes can be identified. Additional information is present in the signal because the amplitude of the resonant frequencies corresponds to the amount of material present at that location.

Chapter 4

Imaging Methods with NMR

Although we are going to deal with only a few examples of the possible imaging methods used in MRI, there is a large number of options for generating images in terms of manipulating field gradients and RF pulses. Imaging techniques in MRI can be classified into four general categories depending on the volume of tissue that is excited or irradiated and from which the signal is received to make an image. Depending on how the MRI scanner is configured, the excited or irradiated volume can be a single point, a line, a plane, or a large volume of tissue. All of these methods produce images that are ultimately resolved into single points or volume elements (voxels), but the way these points are defined and irradiated or excited in the imaging sequence varies. The single-point technique defines the points in the image by exciting and measuring points or voxels one at a time. Three-dimensional reconstruction methods repeatedly excite and measure, and then, using various computer algorithms, calculate the signal contributed by each point or voxel in the object. The type of imaging method used has important consequences for the quality of the ultimate MR image. One of the difficulties in MRI concerns the large amount of background "noise" relative to the MRI signal (signal-to-noise ratio). The signal-to-noise ratio depends on a variety of factors, including the strength of the magnetic field, the total volume of the room-temperature magnet bore, the imaging technique used, and the excitation volume. Most of the intrinsic noise in the MR imaging system is determined by the NMR instrument itself. Because excitation of larger volumes produces larger MRI signals, and because the noise level is determined by the scanner, improvement in the signal-to-noise ratio results when whole-volume excitation methods are employed. On the other hand, as the size of the resolution volume increases with respect to the object size, blurring will decrease contrast in the ultimate image. Thus, when a very small object is scanned with a relatively large resolution volume, although the signal-to-noise ratio increases for the instrument, blurring will decrease spatial resolution in the ultimate image. As we shall see shortly, the FID method provides a stronger signal than do pulse echoes in the spin-echo technique. However spin-echo sequences may actually provide a higher signal-to-noise ratio in the ultimate image by enhancing contrast between adjacent organs with different T_2 relaxation times.

Essentially, the imaging techniques used in MRI involve a series of options regarding the sequencing of either 90° or 180° RF pulses and the timing between the sequences (repetition rate). The options are used to spatially encode and determine different characteristics of tissue, i.e., proton density and T_1 and T_2 relaxation times. The strategies are designed primarily to elicit some aspect of the MRI signal in preference to others with an eye toward a more accurate diagnosis or better contrast or spatial resolution.

Partial-saturation, inversion-recovery, and small-tip-angle methods are used to move the net tissue magnetization into the desired plane, and echo signals are produced by using gradient-recalled echo and spin-echo techniques. These are the most commonly employed imaging methods today. Another method that is commonly used in spectroscopy is called the steady-state-free-precession method or continuous-wave method. In this NMR technique, the magnetic field is periodically tipped by closely pulsed RF excitations. These pulses are short with respect to the T_1 of the sample being irradiated, and in this method sequential FIDs merge and form a continuous NMR signal. A continuous signal has the advantage of providing a steady rather than transient source of energy. However, the nuclei are never allowed to return to equilibrium with the main field, and thus the NMR signal is reduced, but the signal-to-noise ratio is relatively high because it can have a very long duration. RF tissue heating may be a problem, however.

STANDARDIZED IMAGING SEQUENCE

NMR experiments and imaging methods can be thought of in terms of two periods: a period of tissue excitation or preparation, and a period of emission of the absorbed excitation or a period of listening. The way in which these parameters are manipulated is by varying the pulse sequences as follows:

Pulse sequences. Sets of RF (and/or gradient-magnetic-field echoes) pulses and time spacings between these pulses are used in conjunction with gradient magnetic fields and NMR signal reception to produce NMR images.

Interpulse times. Times between successive RF pulses used in pulse sequences are called interpulse times. Particularly important are the inversion time (TI, the time between the 180° and 90° pulses) in inversion-recovery imaging and the time between a 90° pulse and subsequent 180° pulse to produce a spin-echo. This interval will be approximately one-half the spin-echo time (TE). The time between repetitions of pulse sequences is the repetition time (TR) (see Appendix I).

SELECTIVE-EXCITATION IMAGING TECHNIQUES

Single-point, single-line, and single-plane selection techniques. Previously we have seen how it is possible to irradiate a tissue with a broad range of RF waves and with a magnetic-field gradient to determine the position of a given nuclear receiver-transmitter on the basis of its emitted characteristic resonant frequency. Because the resonant frequencies of hydrogen and other nuclear species capable of NMR are known, it is also possible to use a single coherent frequency (as opposed to a broad band) to locate a thin plane of tissue for which the gradient magnetic field and frequency match.

It may be useful to return to the WNMR transmitter in discussing this point. If WNMR transmits only a one-frequency signal (Fig. 3.36, 60″) and similarly tuned receiver-transmitters are aligned in planes, then only a thin plane of the appropriate "tuned" receiver-transmitter antenna will be excited, and our TV receiver will find that only 60″ signals are transmitted from a very thinly defined plane. In NMR imaging we achieve this selectivity of proton receiver-transmitters by applying a gradient magnetic field. If we retain the information from the original plane of excitation, move WNMR perpendicular to the tissue, and again irradiate the tissue with a signal of different frequency, a new plane perpendicular to the first will be the only one tilted 90° by the signal and again subsequently rebroadcasting (transmitting) to our TV receiver on the other side. An observer will then be in a position to define either one of the two planes or define the single receiver-transmitter by the intersection of three planes. In NMR imaging, this arrangement of the receiver-transmitter antenna will be achieved by alternately applying perpendicular gradient magnetic fields. Following a similar procedure for three-dimensional imaging, we can also define a third plane perpendicular to the first two and find the single voxel (volume of tissue) defined by the receiver-transmitter at the exact center of the intersection of the three planes.

By selective excitation in MRI, we can excite only those nuclei (protons) in a thin slice of the body or those in a single line or a single voxel. In NMR this is generally accomplished by applying one gradient during excitation and then applying a second or third gradient perpendicular to it during the readout. In actual practice, the excitation RF pulse is a broadcast of many frequencies, and in effect each proton becomes a small transmitter. The information contained has spatial encoding in the frequency of each signal, and signals from many protons are transmitted at once. The RF signal also has information about the number of proton transmitters and the character of the tissue, as revealed by the amplitude or level of energy. In NMR imaging, selective excitation is accomplished by manipulating the net magnetization vector with the appropriate RF pulse ($90°$ RF$_x$ and $180°$ RF$_x$) to define the plane or line or point of interest.

By using an RF pulse for the appropriate duration and along the appropriate axis, we can actually tip net tissue magnetization through any number of desired degrees of rotation. Essentially, three-dimensional spatial encoding in MRI combines the gradient magnetic field with various degrees of RF pulse rotation to isolate planes, lines, and points of tissue with uniquely oriented magnetic dipoles and net magnetization. If, for example, a given RF pulse tips the net magnetization vector M $90°$ ($90°$ RF$_x$), then a pulse of twice the strength or twice the duration will cause a further displacement of M such that it will lie along the z axis, or a $180°$ shift ($180°$ RF$_x$).

As an example, by combining the techniques of inversion-recovery and gradient manipulation, three-dimensional spatial information can be determined as follows: After a 180° pulse, the net tissue magnetization is directed along the z axis in all volume elements in the tissue (Fig. 4.1). After a period, a 90° RF_x pulse is applied with a z gradient such that only those voxels in a plane parallel to the x–y plane are rotated 90° (Fig. 4.1). As transverse relaxation occurs within the excited 90° RF_x plane, additional x and y gradients are applied to provide spatial information for points within the plane. In voxels outside the excited plane, the magnetization continues to recover along the z axis.

To begin spatial encoding with the spin-echo technique, a magnetic gradient is applied along the y axis (Fig. 4.2). The sample is then exposed to a 90° pulse from an RF coil along the x axis (90° RF_x). Only part of the sample—the stimulated or excited volume—at a specific magnetic field strength will resonate with the exact frequency of the 90° pulse. The magnetization M of the excited volume that was pointing along the z axis is now rotated 90° so that it points along the y axis. As with inversion-recovery, those protons outside the excited volume (i.e., outside the plane parallel to the x–z plane) remain parallel to the z axis. At this point, a magnetic gradient along the z axis is applied, and a 180° RF_x pulse is used to irradiate the tissue (Fig. 4.2). The z gradient again selects only that plane that will respond to the 180° RF_x pulse, which is a plane parallel to the plane x–y. Again, the protons that are outside of the two excited planes remain pointing along the z axis. Only those protons at the intersection of the two excited planes will be pointing in the $-y$ direction and therefore will have a uniquely encoded net magnetization of MRI signal. (Protons in the x–y plane volume excited by the 180° RF_x pulse generally point in the $-z$ direction.)

In the preceding sections we have been developing the concept that one of the most important aspects of MRI is its capacity to yield medical images based on five separate characteristics of tissues. As in CT, a cross-sectional MR image can be produced. That is, an MR image can resolve organ structure on the basis of depth and density of the tissue; another can be created representing the T_1 relaxation-time distribution of the same section; in similar fashion, a third image of the section can be created representing the T_2 relaxation-time distribution; and another MR image sensitive to flow can be reconstructed. The MR signal from anything that is rapidly moving and is taken out of the imaging plane will not be recorded by the RF receiver. Thus, little NMR signal will be obtained from structures involving rapid flow, such as the aorta, whereas slower flow around thrombosis or turbulence from atherosclerotic plaque will produce increased MRI signal. Thus, an image can be created that reflects movement or flow within the cross section. Most MRI today represents an amalgamation of the four parameters, plus chemical shift, that have been blended to best illustrate the anatomy or abnormality with which the radiologist and clinician are concerned.

As discussed in previous sections, a way of categorizing imaging techniques is according to the dimension of the excited volume. Assuming the total imaging volume to be divided into n_x, n_y, and n_z voxels along the three spatial coordinates, then n_x, n_y, and n_z signal elements are required to reconstruct the images within this volume. In the simplest imaging experiment, the signal of each voxel is acquired

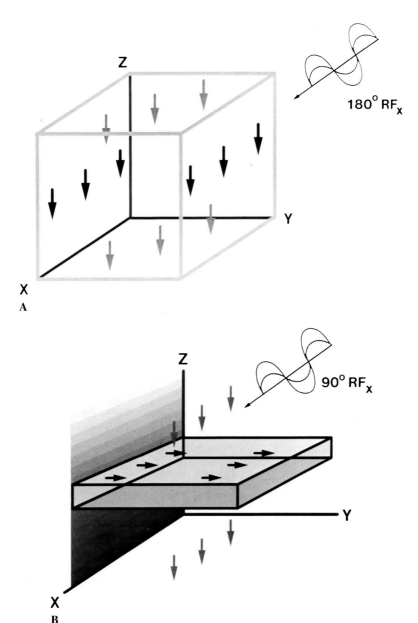

FIG. 4.1. The inversion-recovery imaging sequence can be used to provide spatially encoded information. In this sequence a 180° RF_x pulse inverts the protons in the sample (**A**), and subsequently (**B**) a gradient is applied along the z axis, and a 90° RF_x is pulsed into the tissue at a frequency that is specific for one of the frequency bands identified by the gradient along the z axis. Thus, only those protons in the plane defined by the specific magnetic gradient and matching the frequency of the RF pulse will be shifted 90° along the y axis. Protons outside this plane will continue to be inverted and will slowly relax along the z axis. Thus, the NMR signal obtained will be specific for only the plane defined. A gradient perpendicular to this plane will similarly define a line within that plane, and a plane gradient perpendicular to this can define any voxel desired, and an image can be reconstructed on the basis of this selective information.

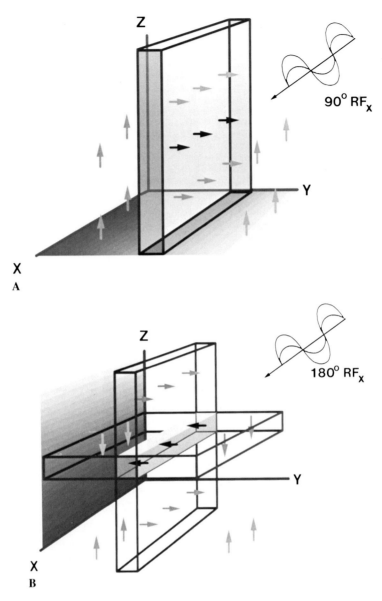

FIG. 4.2. The spin-echo technique can also be used to spatially encode NMR signal infor-mation. In this sequence, a gradient is established along the y axis (**A**), and a 90° RF$_x$ pulse is transmitted to the sample. Again, only those protons precessing at the resonant frequency defined by the gradient will respond to the 90° shift and become oriented along the y axis. Subsequently, the x–y gradient will respond to the 90° shift and become oriented along the y axis. The tissue is irradiated with a 180° RF$_x$ pulse in this second situation (**B**). Again, only those protons in the plane defined by the specific, matching RF frequency and gradient will shift 180°. This results in an inversion of the previously nonexcited nuclei, but those nuclei excited during the 90° RF pulse will now point in the −y direction, thus defining a line. A similar gradient perpendicular to these two can then define a voxel. In practice, these gra-dients are often applied and shifted during both the irradiation and readout phases, but in any event, any voxel in space can be defined using these techniques, and the image can be reconstructed from these individually constructed voxels.

independently. This method, therefore, has been termed the sequential-point or null-point method. Sequential-line and sequential-plane methods are also used. In three-dimensional imaging, the signals of all voxels are observed at the same time. Currently, sequential-point and sequential-line methods have been largely abandoned because signals are gathered from a relatively small number of nuclei. However, planar and volume imaging methods are computationally more demanding. Among the generally adapted planar and volume imaging techniques, three methods have evolved: multiple-angle-projection reconstruction (now rarely used), projection imaging (used in selective-material imaging, as in imaging blood flow), and two- and three-dimensional Fourier transformation.

Back-projection MRI reconstruction was first used by Lauterbur and is currently used widely in CT; however, it is mainly of historical interest in MRI. Briefly, multiple-angle-projection reconstruction was first proposed by Lauterbur and closely resembles X-ray CT reconstruction. It consists of rotating a gradient in small angular displacements to produce, for each angle increment, a projection, or view. The advantage of the multiple-angle-projection reconstruction technique is its relative simplicity and the use of well-established (from X-ray CT) algorithms for image reconstruction. However, in MRI it has the disadvantage of being sensitive to motion artifacts and field inhomogeneity (Fig. 4.3).

Phase-encoding (spin-warp) imaging experiments use a succession of three time periods and magnetic gradients to create a cross-sectional image representing a plane whose picture elements (pixels) are characterized by x and y coordinates. During the first RF pulse, one of the two perpendicular gradients, G_x, is active. This gradient is turned off after t_x sec, and gradient G_y is activated, during which time (t_y) the signal is collected. During the two periods, the magnetization precesses at the frequency determined by the strength of the magnetic field.

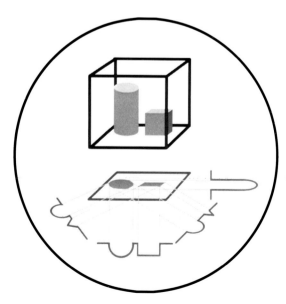

FIG. 4.3. In the filtered back-projection method of image reconstruction, which is the method used in X-ray CT scanning, multiple projections of the desired volume are obtained. The amplitude of the NMR signal is used to assign the number of nuclei present, and the frequency of the signal is used to assign the spatial location. Multiple projections or angles of view are obtained by back-projecting these multiple views. The objects contained within the scanning area can be resolved. In practice, in order to image a matrix of $N \times N$ pixels, N angles of view with N points (detectors) per view are required.

FILTERED BACK-PROJECTION

Zeugmatography as related to NMR imaging was originally described by Lauterbur in 1973. As mentioned in Chapter 3, it implies the yoking together of the magnetic fields and of NMR and electromagnetic waves in the RF range. Essentially, the NMR information is used to produce a "picture" of the internal structures of the human body or any tissue or structure having magnetic nuclei within it.

The technique involves obtaining many projections and is similar to the problem faced by the investigator who has been given the task of determining what, if any, structures have been placed in a room that is surrounded on all four sides by a sheet over which he cannot see. The only tools he is given to solve the problem are a light bulb inside the room that he can move by a remote control and a piece of chalk. His approach in solving this problem is a simplified version of that used in CT and zeugmatography imaging. The investigator walks around the perimeter of the room, always keeping the light bulb against the far wall perpendicular to him and stopping at various points to trace the shadows cast by the objects in the room on the sheet. After outlining all the silhouettes, the investigator draws perpendicular lines from each of the shadows cast on the sheet and projects them back to their point of intersection in the room. From these "back-projections" he constructs his best estimate of the positions and configurations of the objects in the room. Of course, if he takes the time to take more projections, he can come closer to the true configurations and placements of the objects in the room. This principle is equally true for NMR and CT reconstruction techniques; i.e., the more angles of view one obtains, the more accurate the image will be.

In NMR back-projection imaging, as well as in back-projection imaging in CT, the reconstruction problem is similar, except that computers do the work of reconstruction. The technique involves obtaining many projections and then, after some computer filtering to eliminate background noise and then performing other imaging-process techniques, back-projecting the data, i.e., proton-density data, to produce the image.

The first step in this process is to place the object or area of interest within the aperture of the circular magnet of the NMR scanner. A central portion of this aperture is arbitrarily divided up into a grid-like matrix of rectangular cells called voxels that have a finite depth, usually determined by the slice thickness elected for the imaging procedure (voxel = volume element), and a square, arbitrarily defined end surface called the pixel (pixel = picture element). Pixels are so called because they represent in two-dimensional imaging the data obtained from the volume of tissue imaged, and because most of the images are viewed on a TV picture tube or cathode-ray tube (CRT), the pixel usually is the basic element used with most NMR and CT scanning systems.

After the grid-like matrix has been established, multiple projections of an object can be made by changing the direction of the gradient in the x, y, and z planes and back-projecting these data to form an image of the object in cross section, as illustrated in Fig. 4.3. As mentioned previously, the data used to reconstruct the image can involve proton density or T_1 or T_2 relaxation time, or a combination of all three of these parameters. In any event, after many projections are obtained, the computer assigns to each voxel the mean value for the volume of tissue scanned in that element, and this value is then assigned to the pixel for viewing on the CRT.

TWO- AND THREE-DIMENSIONAL FOURIER TRANSFORMATION

We have seen previously how it is possible to encode spatial information by using a magnetic gradient because of the dependence of resonant frequency on regional magnetic field strength. Thus, knowing a given frequency, we are able to assign a position in space to the nuclei emitting that frequency. It is also possible to encode spatial information by making the position in the precessional rotation about the static magnetic field correspond to spatial information.

Let us consider an analogy from baseball. Circumstances arise in which three successive batters get base hits, resulting in A, B, and C being on third, second, and first bases, respectively. Subsequently, batter D also hits a single, advancing A to home for the first run. But using a picture of the diamond for a record, it is difficult to determine if A or E has just scored.

One way to approach this problem is to put oneself in the position of a baseball coach who needs a player to steal bases. The problem is to keep track, in some way, of five baseball players (A to E) who are trying out for the team. The coach finds that all the players have the same running speed and decides to record player performance on baseball-diamond drawings to track player progress around the bases. Although player running speeds cannot be used to determine base-running position, because all players have the same speed, each player's position and base-running ability are represented by each player's rotational progress around the four bases of the diamond. This eliminates the confusion as to whether A or E is up to bat or has just scored the first run. In this method of keeping track of the players, E is assigned the initial starting position zero, D one-quarter, C one-half, B three-quarters, and A one, indicating their progression around the bases (Fig. 4.4). It might also be possible to assign the baseball players positions on the sine wave with a recurring pattern to represent their respective positions. As more runs are scored; the players could be advanced through successive sine-wave cycles (Fig. 4.4).

In NMR imaging, using the method of two-dimensional Fourier transform (2DFT) reconstruction, a set of voxels in an x–y plane is defined with a z gradient. A second gradient applied along the x axis again permits positions along the x axis to be frequency-encoded, and a row of voxels along the y axis can be defined. Up to this time, we have applied no gradient along the y axis, and therefore the precessional frequencies are equal along the y axis. In addition, the precessing magnetization vectors of these tissue voxels remain in phase. In order to assign a unique characteristic to each voxel so that the NMR signal can be immediately assigned to any given voxel in three-dimensional space (thus precluding the necessity for filtered back-projection), a special magnetic gradient can be added along the y axis

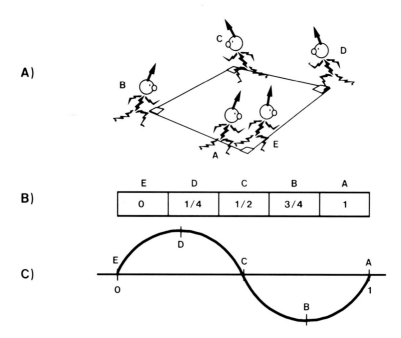

FIG. 4.4. Four baseball players have the same speed; i.e., their frequencies in rounding the bases are identical. Keeping track of their base-running ability by merely monitoring their speed is not satisfactory. One way of approaching this situation is to assign a base-running phase to each player. In this case, as the base runners come up to home plate and begin their cycles around the diamond, runner A, who has just completed one cycle, can be differentiated from runner E, who has yet to begin. Each successive player can then be assigned a value depending on his position in the cycle, and this can be represented by a cycling sine wave (**C**).

specifically to provide phase shifts in the precessing nuclei (Fig. 4.5). The y gradient is applied so that magnetization of the voxel in the strongest field (A) is one cycle ahead of that in the weakest field (E) when the gradient is turned off, at which point this row of voxels will again experience the static magnetic field along the z axis and continue to precess at the same frequency; yet they are out of phase in a predictable way with each other. We can record these phase shifts by using a sine-wave representation, similar to the method used to keep track of the baseball players (Fig. 4.5). Each shift in phase will encode spatial information along the y axis. Imaging requires a sequence of many phases, because the sum of voxels of different phases is all that can be resolved.

TIMING SEQUENCES IN 2DFT

Spin-warp imaging, first proposed by Edelstein and associates, creates a phase twist by varying the timing of gradient and RF pulses to phase-encode spatial information along a preselected axis. In the examples included in this book (Figs. 4.6

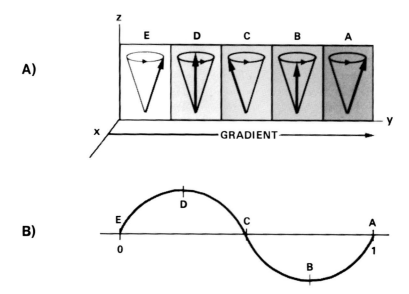

FIG. 4.5. In 2DFT reconstruction, phase encoding of the NMR signal is similar to the phase encoding in Fig. 4.4. For example, a gradient is applied prior to RF tissue irradiation such that all nuclei are precessing at slightly different but defined rates. The gradient is then switched off, and the imaging sequence begins, such that the defined voxels are precessing at the same precessional frequency, but they are out of phase with each other in a defined way. Thus, although the precessional frequency is the same for each voxel, the phase shift represents a specific spatial signature, and this information can be used to reconstruct the image. Timing diagrams are displayed in the following figures in this chapter.

through 4.9), the phase-encoded axes are indicated by G-read. During the initial-pulse portion of the timing sequence, an RF pulse is applied, in this example a 90° RF pulse, and the pulse is made slice-selective by applying a gradient (G-slice) by which the frequency of the RF pulse is matched exactly to the resonant frequency of the protons in the slice. The slice gradient is biphasic to reverse any phase differences created during the G-slice gradient. Following the slice-selective 90° pulse, only protons in the selected slice are excited and are tilted over in the *x–y* plane, where they are still precessing at the resonant frequency.

The 90° selective RF pulse is then followed by a nonselective 180° pulse. The 180° pulse is used to cause a spin-echo in the protons within the excited slice. It is not necessary to make the 180° pulse slice-selective, as only the protons precessing in the *x–y* plane will produce a spin-echo as a result of the 180° pulse. Other protons will merely be inverted, and no signal will be obtained from them. Subsequently, a gradient is applied along the phase-encoded axis (G-phase), and this imparts a characteristic phase signature to each column of protons selected by the G-phase gradient. In the example (Fig. 4.8), clocks, each with a single minute hand, are used to illustrate the various rows and columns of protons being influenced by the phase and frequency gradients. As indicated in the figure, during the phase-encod-

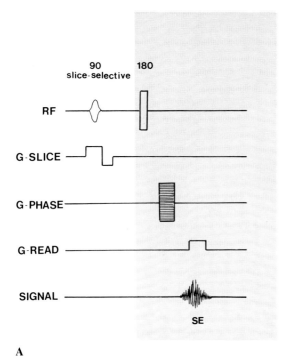

A

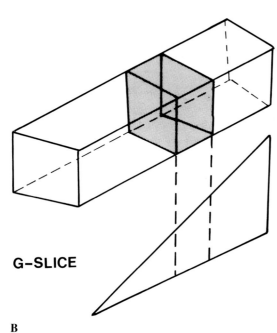

G–SLICE

B

FIG. 4.6. 2DFT imaging: slice selection. The first step in 2DFT imaging is to select the slice to be excited. In this example, an axial section of the rectangle is selected by applying a 90° slice-selective pulse. In these illustrations, RF indicates the RF pulses used in the sequence. G-slice indicates the axis used for slice selection. G-phase indicates the axis along which a phase-encoded gradient is applied. G-read indicates the axis along which the frequency-encoded gradient is applied. The terminology "G-read" indicates that this gradient is applied at the time of signal reception by the receiver RF coil. The signal is indicated along the signal line. Although a FID begins immediately following the 90° RF pulse, it is not indicated in this timing diagram, because this signal is generally ignored in MRI. The 90° slice-selective and G-slice pulses are applied simultaneously and select the plane indicated (**B**). The G-slice gradient is biphasic in order to reverse any phase angle induced in the selected slice during the 90° RF pulse.

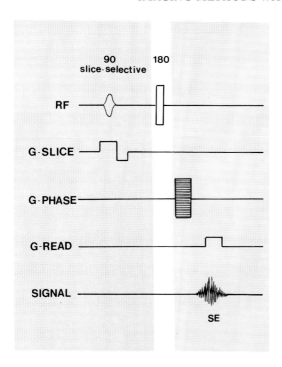

FIG. 4.7. The second step in the 2DFT sequence involves application of a nonselective 180° RF pulse, as indicated in the top RF line. The 180° pulse is used to induce a spin-echo in the excited slice selected during the slice-selective phase. It is not necessary to make this 180° pulse slice-selective, because only those protons precessing in the x–y plane will be induced to rotate 180° and produce a spin-echo.

ing gradient application, the rows of clocks achieve similar phase angles because of application of the phase-encoding gradient. Three rows have been selected here to simplify the illustration, although in clinical practice today, from 128 to 512 rows of specific phase signatures are possible.

During the final period of the imaging sequence, a readout gradient that is frequency-encoded (G-read) is applied at the time when the spin-echo signal is recorded in the receiver antenna. Thus, signal will be received at exactly twice the time interval between the 90° slice-selective pulse and the 180° nonselective pulse. The effect of the G-read is to speed up or slow down the columns of protons selected by the frequency gradient. In the example, the three columns of frequencies have been selected from slowest on the left (hour) through fastest on the right (second). After the G-read gradient has been applied, each voxel has a unique combination of frequency and phase encoding, and by using Fourier transformation we can reconstruct the amplitude (or phase) in a gray-scale or color image.

The major difference between 2DFT and 3DFT imaging is that the slice-selective portion of the imaging sequence is eliminated in 3DFT, and all data are recorded from the entire volume of tissue to be imaged. Slices are selected subsequently by applying a phase-encoding gradient along the third remaining axis such that the final image is composed of individual voxel signatures that have unique phase angles in two dimensions and a unique frequency of precession in the third dimension.

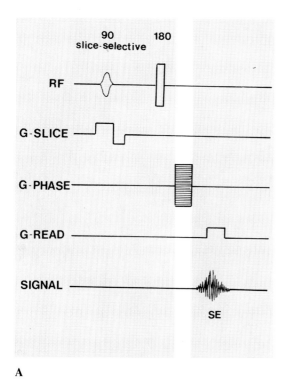

FIG. 4.8. 2DFT phase-encoding step. Protons in the preselected slice are now precessing with identical frequencies, as indicated by the identical minute hands on the clock faces in this diagram (**B**). In other words, all clocks are keeping the same time, and thus their minute hands are all rotating at the same frequency. However, during the phase-encoding portion of this sequence, a phase-encoding gradient (G-phase) selects rows of clocks to accelerate forward (i.e., provide a phase angle or accelerate the minute hands in a predefined manner). The largest gradients in the diagram are applied to the top row, and these have accelerated to the 9:00 position, those in the middle row to the 6:00 position, and those in the bottom row to the 3:00 position. Although three rows and columns are indicated in this diagram, it is possible in current MRI to select from 128 to 512 rows and columns depending on the particular circumstances of the imaging or diagnostic requirements.

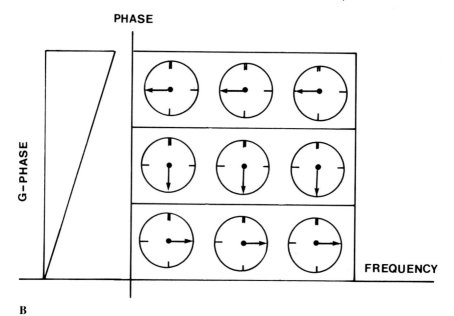

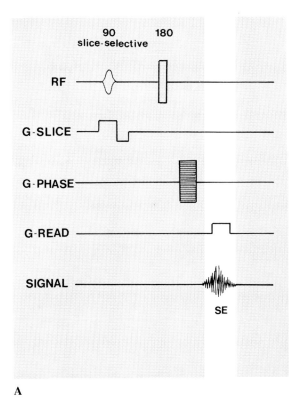

A

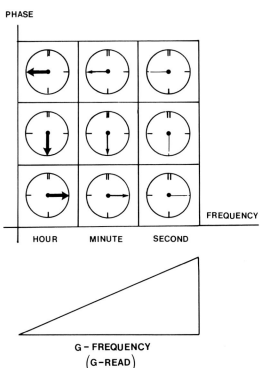

B

FIG. 4.9. 2DFT readout and frequency encoding. A unique signature is applied to each voxel during the frequency-encoding readout phase of the sequence. A gradient is applied in this example so that higher magnetic frequencies occur progressively along the x axis. This gradient has now caused the protons (clocks in this example) to keep different time, or, in other words, to precess at different frequencies. In the illustration, three columns of precessional frequencies have been selected to correspond to an hour hand, minute hand, and second hand on the clock face. Thus, the hour hands move more slowly than the minute hands, etc. Each proton voxel (or clock face in this example) thus has a unique precessional frequency (time-keeping hand) and a unique phase angle (position on the clock face). A Fourier transform operation on both the frequency- and phase-encoded information results in assignment of proton amplitude or magnitude appropriately to each voxel. The signal is read during this time as a spin-echo. The spin-echo signal occurs at exactly twice the time interval between the 90° and 180° RF pulses. At this point, one excitation or imaging sequence has occurred. In order to produce a complete image, it is necessary to repeat the sequence as many times as necessary to reconstruct the data matrix. In this case, we have three columns of frequency-encoded data and three columns of phase-encoded data, and therefore the imaging sequence will have to be repeated three times. Each time the sequence is repeated, a slightly different phase-encoding gradient will be used. A matrix with 128 steps will have to have 128 phase-angle samplings; 256 will require 256, and so on. 3DFT imaging deletes the slice-selective portion of the sequence and irradiates the entire tissue with a 90° pulse. Each slice is then selected with a phase-encoding gradient replacing the G-slice. It is still necessary to repeat the sequence an appropriate number of times to provide the desired matrix size (e.g., 128, 256, or 512).

Chapter 5

MRI Gray Scale: What Does It Mean?

What does the gray scale in an MR image mean? This is one of the most important and most often asked questions by residents and visiting fellows in our MRI programs. Let us begin with a rule of thumb (visual–cluster–analysis) before exploring this complex topic in more depth. First we must organize the MRI study so that we are sure how the study was performed (i.e., sequences used, orthogonal views, etc.). We place short-TR/TE studies first, long-TR/TE studies next, and then any special studies such as small-tip-angle/gradient-recalled echo sequences, short-TI studies, etc. Using our knowledge of normal anatomy and the patient's history, we identify tissue such as fat, fatty marrow, cortical bone, tendon, air, surgical clips, muscle, liquids (e.g., urine in bladder, or renal pelvis, cerebrospinal fluid, etc.), blood (normal uterine cavity), and flowing blood in arteries and veins. Without making any attempt to further understand the exact sequences used, we follow each tissue through each imaging sequence to determine the changes in gray scale in each succeeding study. Next we inspect all tissue types to confirm that they are homogeneous and that there are no uncharacteristic gray-scale readings in any of the images. Next we compare any unknown structures with the known tissues to see if a gray-scale pattern matches the unknown. An angiomyolipoma of the liver will appear different than normal liver, will not be confused with a liver cyst because it does not "perform" like the bladder or renal pelvis, and will be suggested because the MRI gray-scale findings will be duplicated by fat and muscle intensities. A liver hemangioma will look like blood clots or slow blood flow in veins (ascending lumbar, hemorrhoidal, etc.). Thus, using the tissues present within the image, a considerable amount of information can be obtained from the gray-scale images without knowing much detail about why they look as they do. Loops of bowel can be confusing; however, the MRI study takes approximately an hour to complete, and loops of bowel should move between the times the three orthogonal views are taken. This is not characteristic of solid neoplasms, abscesses, etc.

Part of the confusion regarding MRI gray-scale interpretation is possibly related to one's previous experience with CT scanning. CT scanning, as it is practiced clinically, involves using X-rays to measure the linear-attenuation coefficient of X-rays in tissue, assigning that number to an arbitrary integer scale (usually $\pm$ 1,000), and then, by using window and level settings, assigning a gray (white to black) scale to the entire range, or perhaps a subdivision of the CT number range. Once one point of this scale is fixed, i.e., if cortical bone is assigned + 1,000 on the CT number scale, then all tissues are linearly related to that point according to their densities. Images may be made lighter or darker by using the appropriate window and level settings; however, all tissue intensities are changed proportionately.

One of the difficulties in MR imaging is that the image is based on a number of parameters, and depending on which parameter is emphasized or selected, tissues may show changes in their relative positions on the gray scale. One of the most striking examples of this phenomenon is the black appearance of moving blood in the aorta on a conventional spin-echo image, but a white appearance on a gradient-recalled echo sequence. Cortical bone, on the other hand, appears black in both images.

In order to understand the significance of the gray-scale assignment (or the color assignment, for that matter) it is necessary to understand the fundamental determinants of MRI contrast. We can divide the determinants into sequence (scanner-related factors) and tissue (intrinsic biochemistry of the tissue) determinants. Tissue MR signal determinants involve nuclear density. T_1 and T_2 relaxation parameters, tissue motion or flow, and chemical shift. Factors intrinsic to the scanner itself involve imaging sequences, e.g., the choice between RF or gradient pulses, and timing decisions, e.g., choices between TR, TE, TI, etc. The sequence factors can be utilized to elucidate or emphasize various tissue factors. For example, proton-nuclear-density images can be obtained by using very long TR and very short TE pulses. In such a sequence, gray matter will be seen to be of higher signal intensity than white matter because of the fact that its proton nuclear density is slightly higher.

TR AND TE DETERMINANTS OF THE MRI GRAY SCALE

NMR experiments or imaging methods can be thought of in terms of two periods: a period of tissue excitation or preparation, and a period of emission or a period of listening. The methods by which these parameters are manipulated are as follows:

Pulse sequences. Sets of RF (and/or gradient) magnetic-field pulses and time spacings between these pulses are used in conjunction with gradient magnetic fields and NMR signal reception to produce NMR images.

Interpulse times. Interpulse times are the times between successive sets of RF pulses used in pulse sequences. Particularly important are the inversion time (TI) in inversion-recovery and the time between a 90° pulse and the subsequent 180° pulse to produce a spin-echo. This interval will be approximately one-half the spin-echo time (TE). The time between repetitions of pulse sequences is the repetition time (TR) (see Appendix I).

An NMR image is extremely dependent on the techniques employed in administering the various RF pulses. Variations in TR and TE can increase the contrast between tissues by exploiting differences between their relaxation rates. If we consider adjusting the sequence by shortening the TR, we begin to decrease the signal coming from those tissues with longer T_1 values, while those with shorter T_1 values (i.e., those T_1 values shorter than the TR) maintain their signal intensities. In the spin-echo technique, by lengthening the TE or using chains of 180° pulses (although the spin-echo amplitudes of all tissues decline), those tissues with longer T_2 values maintain their signal intensities, whereas short-T_2 signal intensities fall off rapidly. Absolute measurement of T_1 and T_2 relaxation times is very dependent on the equipment and field strengths, i.e., B_0 used; however, as a general approximation, in comparing muscle and fat, the T_1 and T_2 values for muscle are 0.7 sec and 32 msec, respectively, and for fat, 0.3 sec and 50 msec, at 1 T.

As we adjust the NMR imaging instrumentation, fat will be seen as brighter (whiter) than muscle when using a short-TR or a long-TE technique because of the shorter T_1 and longer T_2 in fat tissue. In NMR imaging, varying the TR and TE (T_1 and T_2 selection) parameters can also selectively enhance the contrast between tissues. In a comparison of fat and muscle, lengthening the T_2 (i.e., TE) parameters will decrease the absolute T_2 signal intensities, but the contrast between the tissues will increase. Thus, obtaining NMR images at several instrument TR and TE settings is advisable because the densities of pathological lesions may blend with those of surrounding normal tissues and may be missed if only one setting is used.

TR

In MRI, adjustment of TR, which separates the two periods of RF-pulse excitation and emission, can have an important impact on the quality and diagnostic utility of an NMR image. Following the 90° pulse, if the TR is made too short relative to the length of T_1, there will be a decrease in the initial signal amplitude observed (Figs. 5.1 and 5.2). This occurs because insufficient time is allowed for longitudinal relaxation, and M_z is not fully recovered to its equilibrium value. From this perspective, two tissues being scanned using a fixed 90° RF_x repetition rate, but with markedly different T_1 values, will have different NMR signals—a very intense signal if T_1 is short, and a somewhat less intense signal if T_1 in the second tissue is relatively longer (Fig. 5.2). This principle can be exploited by NMR imaging technology to produce contrast differences among tissues based on differences in relaxation rates. When TR is long relative to T_1, a maximum signal amplitude is obtained, i.e., A_1 in Figs. 5.1 and 5.2. However, if we shorten the TR and do not allow complete relaxation, we notice a decrease in the initial signal amplitude of the ensuing FID (A_2 in Fig. 5.2).

TE

Tissue contrast differences can be increased based on their differing T_2 relaxation times by varying TR times or using multiple-echo techniques (see Appendix I).

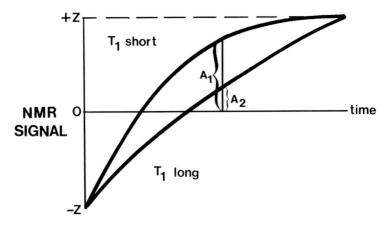

FIG. 5.1. The repetition rate or TR has a marked effect on the NMR signal obtained from two tissues with varying T_1 relaxation times. A tissue with a short T_1 will have a maximum amplitude (A_1); however, a tissue with a T_1 that is longer will result in a much reduced amplitude (A_2). This effect is seen in an NMR image as a decrease in NMR signal or a shift toward the black end of the gray scale. A very long TR interval will essentially remove any T_1 information from the image. Proton-density images take advantage of this fact by using long TR without an echo or with a very short TE to severely restrict any T_2-relaxation information in the image. T_1 also increases with field strengths, B_0.

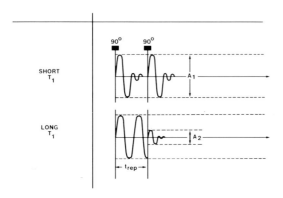

FIG. 5.2. See Fig. 5.1.

Tissues with differing T_2 relaxation times, as illustrated in Fig. 5.3, will characteristically show increasing contrast differences as TE is lengthened until both are completely relaxed. Knowing the optimal period to exploit these differences is impossible prior to imaging, and therefore a multiple-echo technique can "sample" these differences. The price paid for this increased information is in longer imaging times.

The T_2 relaxation time is important when using the spin-echo technique in NMR imaging. TE and tissue T_2 have little effect on the amplitude (signal intensity) of an FID following a 90° pulse. However, TR and the length of T_1 can have a significant effect on the intensity of the spin-echo. If the TR is shortened so that net tissue magnetization M_z is not completely reestablished, then the z-oriented magnetization

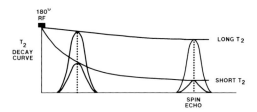

FIG. 5.3. In imaging sequences using the spin-echo technique, although the T_2 values for all tissues will decrease following the 180° RF pulse, those with longer T_2 values will demonstrate stronger NMR signals than a tissue with a shorter T_2, resulting in improved contrast enhancement and tissue lesion detectability. This effect is produced in the MR image by using long TE intervals. Maximum T_2 weighting of the image is produced by using long TR intervals to allow complete T_1 relaxation and then using long-TE or multiple-echo techniques.

at the beginning of the next spin-echo sequence (90° RF_x) will start out weaker, and the resultant M_{xy} and thus the spin-echo will have less signal intensity as well. In other words, a short TR interval will tend to decrease the intensity of the following spin-echo signal, all other factors being held constant.

SEQUENCE DETERMINANTS OF IMAGE CONTRAST

Table 5.1 should be used as a guide in evaluating the images in Fig. 5.4. These midline 1.5-T sagittal MR images of the brain, all performed on the same subject on the same sequential series of scans, have been chosen to demonstrate the effects on image contrast and spatial resolution as the factors are adjusted. The base-line imaging sequence for comparison involves a partial-saturation technique, with TR = 400 msec, TE = 25 msec, the number of averages being two, a matrix of 256 × 256, and a 5-mm slice thickness with a 20% gap between slices. From this basic sequence and timing selection, the following are illustrated: TR values varying from 2,500 to 200 msec; a four-echo spin-echo sequence with TE values equal to 25, 50, 75, and 100 msec; 3-mm and 20-mm slice thicknesses; no gap between contiguous slices; six averages; a 12-cm field of view; and a matrix of 128 × 256. A horizontal RF artifact is present on some of the images. Figure 5.5 demonstrates a full TR/TE sequence at the level of the pulmonary artery for comparison.

FACTORS AFFECTING TISSUE SIGNAL INTENSITY
AND GRAY-SCALE IMAGING

The parameters that affect tissue contrast include the following: solid or liquid state, water content, lipid content and type, perturbed water motion, macromolecular motion, and paramagnetic species (e.g., contrast agents). In addition, there are extraneous factors that can affect tissue contrast, including patient dehydration, drugs, diet, and temperature. Tissue relaxation changes of as much as 20% have been associated with commonly prescribed medications, and dietary manipulations

TABLE 5.1. *Effects of changing sequence parameters*

Parameter	Contrast-to-noise ratio[a]	Signal-to-noise ratio[b]	Spatial resolution[c]	Acquisition time[d]
TR(+)	0[e]	+	0	+
TR(−)	0	−	0	−
TE(+)	0	−	0	0
TE(−)	0	+	0	0
Slice thickness(+)	+	+	f	0
Slice thickness(−)	−	−	f	0
Interslice distance(+)	+	+	0	0
Interslice distance(−)	−	−	0	0
FOV(+)	+	+	−	0
FOV(−)	−	−	+	0
NEX(+)	+	+	0	+
NEX(−)	−	−	0	−
256 to 128	+	+	−	−
128 to 256	−	−	+	+

[a]Contrast-to-noise ratio: the difference in regional signal intensities in the image divided by the amount of noise. Contrast is the difference in signal level between two adjacent anatomic regions.
[b]Signal-to-noise ratio: the overall signal divided by the background noise.
[c]Spatial resolution: the distance between two points at which one can distinguish the points as being separate.
[d]To calculate acquisition time: total acquisition time* = (TR) × (acquisition matrix) × (2) × (no. of signal averages) × no. of slices. *For single-slice (2D) and volumetric acquisition. Total acquisition time for interleaved, multislice acquisition can be calculated by keeping number of slices = 1.
[e]0 = not applicable; + = factor increase; − = factor decrease.
[f]Partial-volume-averaging effect.
Note: TE/TE does influence image contrast but this is a function of tissue relaxation and not a scanner determined factor.

involving potassium deficiency or high-cholesterol diets have resulted in as much as a 10% change in tissue relaxation.

Physical state can have significant effects on T_1 and T_2 relaxation times. T_1 is much longer for solids than for liquids. In an external magnetic field, as we have seen previously, protons align parallel and antiparallel with the imposed magnetic field. This process of alignment occurs by molecular thermal interaction; i.e., molecules within the sample collide or interact with each other, thus transferring energy. In solids (which, in general, can be thought of as crystalline lattices), molecules are relatively fixed and do not frequently collide with each other, thereby transferring energy and facilitating proton realignment in the field. T_1 is also called *spin-lattice relaxation* (spin, because of the spinning proton; lattice, because of the physical matrix of the molecule in the sample). As mentioned earlier, it is also often called *longitudinal relaxation* because of the longitudinal orientation with the z axis.

T_2 is much shorter for solids than for liquids. Briefly, solids (e.g., cortical bone) have relatively fixed molecules with relatively fixed magnetic fields, and these cause significant local variations in the value of the magnetic field around any given proton. In a liquid (e.g., soft tissue), the local magnetic fields from neighboring molecules fluctuate rapidly as the molecules move about, and the end result contributes little to the net magnetic field at any point.

In solids, the molecular structure tends to be fixed, and their associated magnetic fields are fixed as well. These local inhomogeneities are significant and cause significant internal magnetic-field effects, especially when the opposing magnetic fields are pointed in the opposite or unaligned direction. Thus, the magnetic-magnetic interaction, or the spin-spin interaction, is quite significant in solids, and T_2 is very short. In a liquid, however, molecules are free to move rapidly, and their net local magnetizations average very quickly to a small value (Fig. 5.6). Magnetic-magnetic or spin-spin interactions are not very significant. Consequently, for liquids, the internal fields are weaker, and T_2 encounters less dephasing magnetic influence, and thus T_2 is longer. Again, as the transverse M_{xy} component decays, the longitudinal component is growing at a rate T_1 because of thermal collisions. Therefore, T_2 is often referred to as the transverse (transverse to the external magnetic field), spin-spin, or proton-proton (magnetic-field-to-magnetic-field interaction) relaxation time.

Because solid tissues and other solid specimens have fixed, static internal magnetic fields that cause variations in the local magnetic field, there are local variations in proton resonant frequencies, and the FID for solids is composed of many sine waves of differing frequencies. Because they quickly get out of phase, the corresponding FID curve, in the time domain, is short (short T_2). For pure liquids, the effect of internal magnetic fields is much less, and the proton resonant frequency is determined almost entirely by the external magnetic field. Thus, there is a narrow band of resonant frequencies shared by all the protons in the excited region. They remain in phase, and therefore the FID for liquids is long. For solids having an FID composed of sine waves of many frequencies, in the frequency domain the frequency spectrum is broad. For liquids, the range of frequencies (or the width of the frequency spectrum) is quite narrow. This is demonstrated in Fig. 5.7, where the amplitude of the sine waves that make up the FID is plotted against the respective frequency. The resultant peak is broad-based for solids and narrow for liquids.

The key to understanding tissue MRI contrast as determined by T_1 and T_2 relaxation phenomena lies in understanding the relationships among tissue water content, tissue water motion, sizes and types of macromolecules (lipid or protein), and type of binding between tissue water and tissue macromolecules. The presence of paramagnetic agents can also have a significant impact on tissue relaxation parameters. The difficulty in utilizing each of these parameters in clinical MRI is further compounded by the fact that interaction between tissue water and tissue macromolecules can be characterized by either fast or slow exchange, as well as by the amount of cross-relaxation (the reciprocal influences of water and macromolecular relaxation rates) and the type of rotation or tumbling action to which the water and macromolecules are subjected. MRI interpretation depends on an understanding of the importance of these biochemical factors with respect to various diagnostic situa-

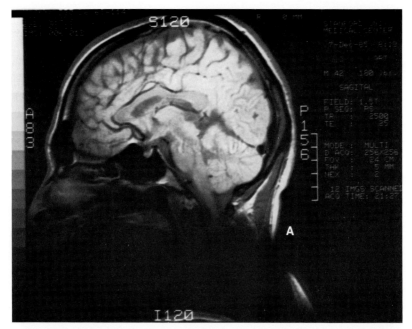

A

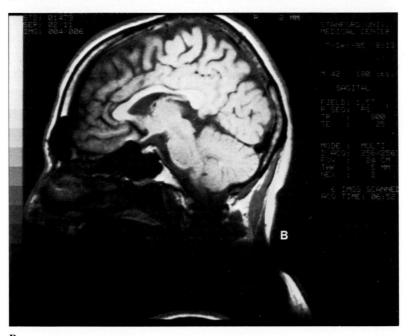

B

FIG. 5.4. This series of sagittal brain MRI studies shows selected slices from multiple scanning sequences taken at the same sagittal level through the brain. This series illustrates the effects of changing various scanning-sequence options when programming the MR scanner. The images should be compared for the indicated effects on image contrast and signal-to-noise ratio from Table 5.1. The scanning parameters used are indicated on the individual images.

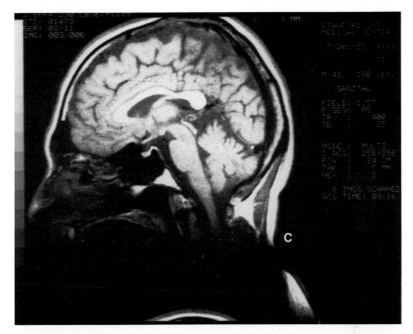

C

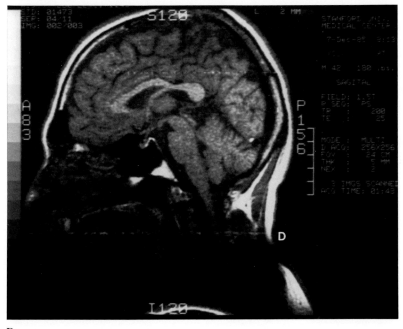

D

FIG. 5.4. (*continued*). Illustrated are effects on image contrast from changing TR values (**A–D**, 2500-260), TE values (**E–H**, 2560/25–100), number of excitations, scanning matrix, slice thickness, skip interval, and field of view (**I–N**). The TR series represents a spectrum from a balanced, mainly proton-weighted image in **A** through a significant decline in signal intensity due to the short TR interval in **D** (Tr = 200 msec). The TE series (**E–H**), using a long Tr value of 2,500 msec, should be compared with the partial-saturation technique illustrated in **A**.

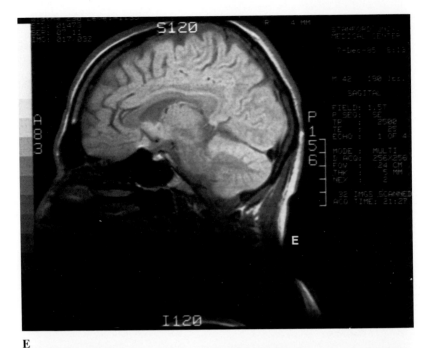

E

F

FIG. 5.4. (*continued*). Tissues with relatively long T_2 values (i.e., CSF) are seen as high signal intensities in image **H,** whereas a proton-density image is seen in image **E.** Increasing the number of excitations increases the contrast-to-noise ratio, signal-to-noise ratio, and acquisition time. This is illustrated by comparing images **I** (NEX = 6) and **C** (NEX = 2). Changing the matrix from 256 × 256 to 256 × 128 increases the contrast-to-noise ratio and signal-to-noise ratio and decreases spatial resolution and acquisition time because of the larger voxels used in the 256 × 128 technique (image **J** compared with image **C**).

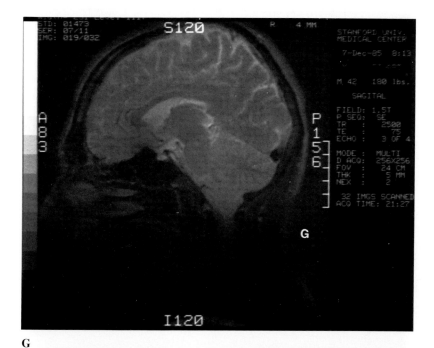

G

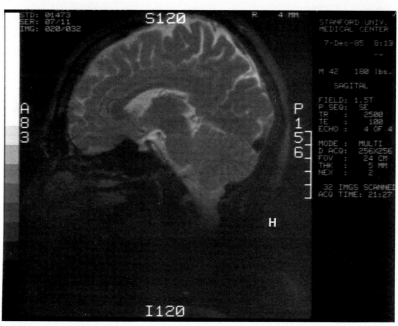

H

FIG. 5.4. (*continued*). Decreasing the slice thickness produces a smaller voxel size and results in decreased contrast-to-noise and signal-to-noise ratios. Spatial resolution is improved because of the smaller slice thickness; however, the resulting image has considerably higher background noise (image **K** compared with image **C**).

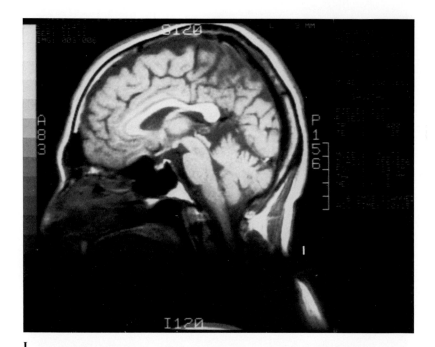

I

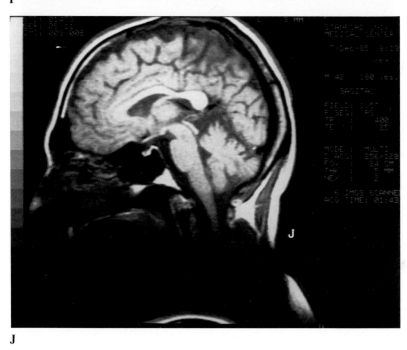

J

FIG. 5.4. (*continued*). Decreasing the interslice interval to zero is illustrated in image **L,** which should be compared with image **K.** The use of contiguous slices in **L** causes cross-relaxation effects between slices and results in decreases in contrast-to-noise and signal-to-noise ratios. The use of a large slice thickness (*M*) similarly increases voxel size and therefore results in increased contrast-to-noise and signal-to-noise ratios.

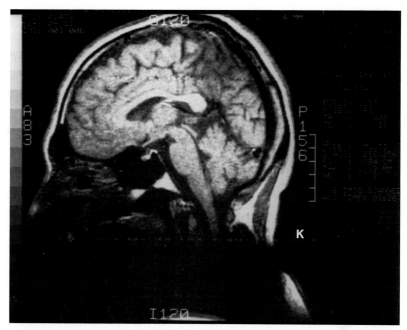

K

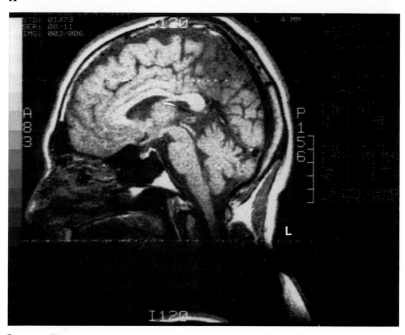

L

FIG. 5.4. (*continued*). Partial-volume effects are increased, and thus spatial resolution is decreased. However, comparison between images **M** and **L** illustrates the difference between 3-mm and 20-mm slice thicknesses. Isolated comparisons between different fields of view are somewhat difficult because of the artifacts induced by this technique: aliasing (*large arrows*), and, incidentally, also some RF artifact best seen in these sequences (*small arrows*).

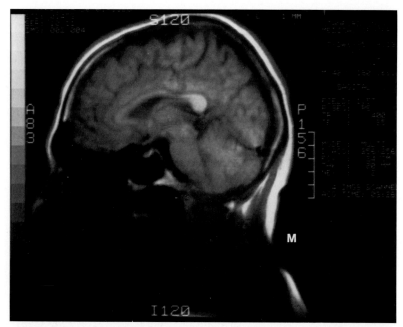

M

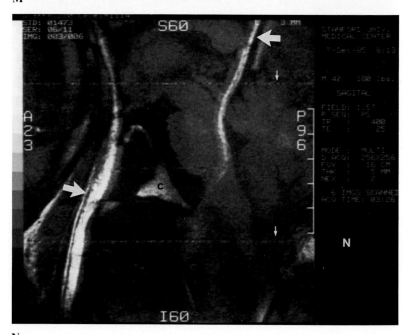

N

FIG. 5.4. (*continued*). The marrow within the clivus is marked for anatomic reference (c). Decreasing the field of view decreases contrast-to-noise and signal-to-noise ratios and increases spatial resolution. Comparison of image N_1 (FOV = 16) with image **C** illustrates this effect.

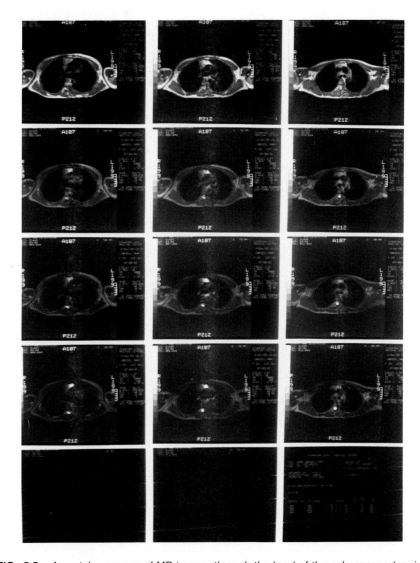

FIG. 5.5. An axial sequence of MR images through the level of the pulmonary artery in a patient with Hodgkin's disease of the anterior mediastinum. The images illustrate the complete set of effects of varying both TR and TE intervals on the tissues at this level. TR values increase from left to right (400, 800, and 2,000 msec), and the echo sequence progresses from top to bottom (25/50/75/100). Thus, short-TR/TE sequences are best illustrated in the upper-left-hand corner, and long-TR/TE sequences are best illustrated in the lower-right-hand corner. Note that fat has a relatively high signal intensity with the short TR/TE intervals because of its relatively short T_1 relaxation time. The anterior mediastinal Hodgkin's disease also yields a relatively high signal in this image. Although overall signal intensity drops off, a cystic collection within the tumor is best seen in the longer-TR/TE sequences. Note that the CSF has its highest intensity in these images as well.

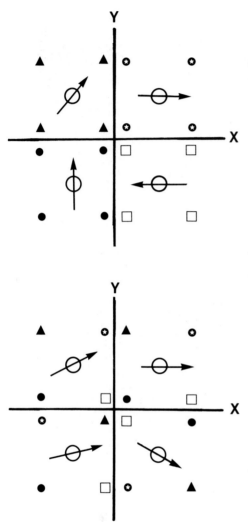

FIG. 5.6. One way to conceptualize the effects of magnetic regional inhomogeneities within tissue on T_2 relaxation times is to use the illustration in the top of this figure representing fixed areas of differing magnetic fields indicated by the four symbols in the four quadrants. This illustration simulates the conditions existing within a tissue, such as muscle, with large relatively fixed tissue molecules and long, correlation times (t_c). Four individual protons are illustrated. The protons precessing coherently following a 90° RF pulse will result in the net magnetization M of the tissue that has been illustrated in many of the previous figures. As the protons spin, they encounter relatively significant fixed areas of magnetic inhomogeneity and experience rapid dephasing and short T_2 relaxation (i.e., rapid loss of M in the x–y plane). If these centers of magnetic inhomogeneity are allowed to move around freely within the tissue, as illustrated in the lower portion of the figure, each proton encounters a more homogeneous type of local magnetic field. Random spin-spin interactions still account for regional precessional frequency differences; however, the differences have been markedly reduced by the more even distribution of the regional magnetic dipoles. In this tissue, which might represent a liquid, T_2 relaxation is much longer because each individual precessing proton encounters a more homogeneous magnetic field than in the example above. T_2 is longer because phase coherence is maintained longer. A similar condition would result if molecular tumbling (T_c) was very fast and much greater than the resonant frequency established by the MR scanner.

tions. For example, NMR signals in the presence of conditions such as dehydration or anasarca depend on the water content of tissue and electrolyte imbalance, and immature cells can be detected on the basis of the relaxation times, as influenced by water content, macromolecular motion, and perturbed water motion. Obesity, muscular dystrophies, and aging are influenced by the tissue lipid content, and the MRI signal is dependent on water content and release of paramagnetics (Fe^{3+}) as hemoglobin passes from the oxyhemoglobin to the deoxyhemoglobin to the methemoglobin state.

Another source of difficulty in understanding tissue characteristics that determine

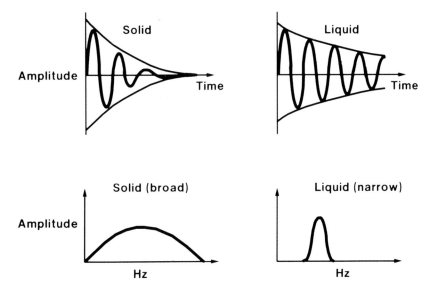

FIG. 5.7. Physical state has a significant effect on T_2 relaxation time. T_2 relaxation occurs by magnetic interaction of protons. Solids have fixed internal magnetic fields that cause variation in the local magnetic field, and therefore precessing protons rapidly dephase, and the FID for solids is composed of many sine waves of differing (broad) frequencies, and the T_2 relaxation time is short. In liquids, internal magnetic fields are not static, and the internal fields quickly sum to zero, having much less effect on the precessing protons. Therefore, the frequency band of precessing protons is narrow, and the relaxation time is long. These are significant considerations, because variations in relaxtion time have significant effects on NMR image contrast.

the gray scale observed on MR images is that the dominance of any of these interactions is field-dependent. For example, at very low field strengths (proton Larmor frequencies of 0.1 MHz), macromolecules dominate organ relaxation times. At this field strength, the relaxation rate for the liver is considerably higher (liver appears white) than that for adipose tissue because the correlation time for the proteins within the liver is closer to the Larmor frequency than that of the smaller fat macromolecules. However, at higher field strengths (proton Larmor frequency of 50 MHz), the relaxation rate for fat is greater (fat appears white) than that for liver because at this higher field strength it is the water molecules within the liver that are predominantly controlling the observed relaxation rate, and because these molecules are considerably smaller and therefore are rotating considerably faster than the resonant frequency of the scanner, the somewhat larger fat molecules have a faster relaxation time. Even though this key to understanding tissue contrast parameters is complex, it is well worth understanding, because it is at the level of molecular biology that MRI has the potential for early diagnosis and treatment of human disorders.

As reviewed previously, the gray scale depicted in MRI is related to a combination of factors that include the density of the nuclear species, T_1 and T_2 relaxation characteristics, motion or flow, and the chemical-shift phenomenon. In this section we shall focus primarily on T_1 and T_2 relaxation times as determinants of image contrast. It is, of course, possible to image nuclear density. For example, by using a TR of 2,400 msec, relative signal intensities progressing from highest to lowest nuclear density can be assigned to cerebrospinal fluid (CSF), gray matter, and white matter, respectively (CSF 100%, gray matter 94%, white matter 80%). The use of motion or flow in producing MR images is discussed in the section on blood flow in Chapter 6. The ability to weight MR images for relaxation parameters is relatively straightforward: T_1 weighting is obtained by using a short-TR and short-TE pulsing sequence, and T_2 weighting is obtained by using a long-TR and long-TE pulsing sequence.

The key to understanding tissue relaxation is in understanding the tumbling or rotational correlation time (t_C) for the molecules within the tissue being imaged (Fig. 5.8). Rotational correlation time can be thought of as the average speed of

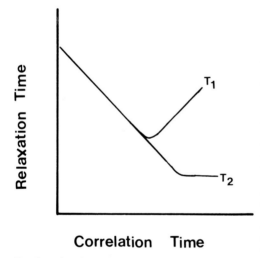

Correlation   Time

FIG. 5.8. Correlation time (t_C). The schematic log-log plot illustrates the effect of molecular tumbling or correlation time on T_1 and T_2 relaxation. Correlation time generally increases with molecular size. Correlation time increases from left to right. Small molecules with molecular weights less than 200 are represented on the left side of the graph, and slower correlation times for molecules with molecular weights greater than 1,000 are represented on the right. Very small molecules can tumble (or rotate) very rapidly and thus are rotating well above the resonant frequency of the protons within those molecules. As molecular size, increases, however, the spinning (or tumbling) of the molecules slows down and begins to approach the resonant frequency of the protons. A minimum, or the shortest, T_1 relaxation time occurs when the correlation time of the molecule is relatively close to the resonant frequency of the protons within that molecule ($t_C = 1/\omega_0$, or correlation time = 1/resonant frequency). T_1 and T_2 changes are similar up to this point. However, as molecular tumbling slows further, fewer molecular collisions (or thermal interactions) occur within the sample, and T_1 relaxation times begin to increase again. T_2 relaxation, however, depends on the amount of magnetic inhomogeneity within the sample. As molecules become larger, their ability to diffuse (or move through the tissue) is decreased, and therefore focal areas of magnetic inhomogeneity result. At a certain molecular size, the tissue essentially becomes solid with respect to T_2 relaxtion and approaches a limiting value or plateau that is characteristic of a completely rigid, solid lattice. Thus, a liquid such as urine in the bladder has a relatively long T_1 and a relatively long T_2, therefore yielding low-intensity signals on short-TR/TE images, but high-intensity signals on long-TR/TE images, whereas muscle yields signals of relatively low intensity on both short-TR/TE and long-TR/TE sequences because the correlation time of the molecules in the tissue is relatively high, resulting in short T_2 relaxation times, but long T_1 relaxation times.

molecular tumbling for any given population of molecules (e.g., water, fat, proteins). Because resonant frequency is determined by B_0, the static field strength of the magnet being used selects the resonant frequency of the system, and it is only that population of molecules tumbling at the resonant frequency of the system that will interact and produce relaxation within the tissues. The reason molecular tumbling influences relaxation rates is because of its effect on dipole interactions. The magnetic field experienced by a proton is the sum of the external magnetic field B_0 and the magnetic field it experiences from other neighboring protons. This additional field flux is approximately ± 10 G (dipole-dipole interaction for the two protons in water) and can cause the proton to vary its resonant frequency by approximately 10^5 Hz. Under these conditions, complete transverse dephasing occurs in approximately 10^{-5} sec; in other words, any large molecule that has slowed down to a rotational frequency of around 10^5 rotations per second will appear to be a solid in NMR experiments. This is a general explanation of relaxation in the theory of Bloembergen, Purcell, and Pound (BPP) (Fig. 5.8).

T_2 relaxation times decrease and then approach a limiting value as one moves from small molecules (fast molecular tumbling) through viscous liquids to solid substances, whereas T_1 relaxation decreases to a minimum and then increases again for solid materials. In body tissues, water, with a molecular weight of 18, has a very fast correlation time (10^{-12} sec), whereas lipids have a molecular weight of approximately 1,000 have correlation times of 10^{-9}, and aqueous proteins have relatively slow correlation times greater than 10^{-9} sec.

The correlation time and relaxation time for water in tissue are directly related to the type of water bonding. Bulk water, with generalized hydrogen bonding, has the shortest correlation time (10^{-12} sec). Structured water, or water that is loosely bound to macromolecules, has a slightly longer correlation time. Water bound to hydrophilic sites on macromolecules has the next longest, and so-called superbound water, held very closely to macromolecules, performs much like a solid (correlation time $>10^{-5}$ sec) (terminology developed by G. Fullerton and associates). Thus, increasing temperature causes increasing T_1 values, because the increased temperature tends to break up hydrogen bonding in the water and therefore allows faster molecular tumbling. Similarly, moving from a nonviscous to a more viscous liquid causes a decrease in correlation. And up to the point where $t_C = 1/\omega_0$, shorter T_1 relaxation times occur. To extend this general principle, any process that tends to increase the binding (or structuring) of water within a relevant range tends to increase the relaxation rate or decrease the relaxation time.

Another important influence on tissue proton relaxation times is the cross-relaxation process by which water protons and protons within the macromolecule influence their respective relaxation rates. This generally occurs in poorly hydrated tissues such as liquids with high solute concentrations (such as proteinaceous pleural effusions or tissues such as collagen). Because of this phenomenon, the correlation time or molecular tumbling of the protein itself can influence proton relaxation. It should be borne in mind, again, that these relationships are field-dependent, so that there is greater differential effect on T_1 relaxation at lower field strengths than at higher field strengths.

Because bound water and structured water generally tend to have slower correlation times and in the proper B_0 field strength generally have shorter relaxation times and higher relaxation rates, as the amount of solute per unit of water increases, so does the relaxation rate. Tissues that have a higher solute-to-water ratio therefore, will have shorter relaxation times. Thus, T_1 for plasma is greater than that for red blood cells because of the lower solute concentration in plasma, and relaxation rates increase linearly with hematocrit because of the increasing amount of solute contained within the red blood cells.

The diffusion rate of water is considerably greater than required to move beyond the diameter of the typical living cell during a NMR experiment, and measured tissue relaxation times therefore reflect the proportionate amount of time water is spending in the various intracellular and extracellular compartments. This offers the attractive possibility of characterizing tissues on the basis of their average relaxation times, and this phenomenon serves as the basis for the hope of being able to characterize neoplastic tissues, because their intracellular and extracellular compartments are, in some instances, quite different from those in normal tissue. Finally, in further compounding this complex situation, a tissue such as fat undergoes slow fat–water exchange, and in certain tissues such as collagen, water molecules are not free to rotate isotropically, and therefore the orientations of these types of tissues to the external magnetic field can greatly influence relaxation parameters.

Thus, the determinants of tissue relaxation times are very complex. The gray-scale assignment of relaxation times will depend greatly on the imaging sequence selected and the tissue being evaluated. CSF has prolonged relaxation times (T_1 and T_2) because it is a liquid with rapidly tumbling small molecules and bulk water. It appears dark on short-TR images and white on long-TE images. White matter has large myelin molecules and appears white on short-TR sequences and darker on long-TE sequences. With the exception of cortical bone, calculi, and metallic clips, most body tissues can be thought of as liquids with various-size molecules dissolved or suspended within them. Disease states often are associated with increased water (i.e., edema), and this increase in water, in general, increases relaxation times (T_1 and T_2).

Many conditions tend to cause similar changes in both T_1 and T_2, but T_1 and T_2 are often inversely related to image contrast if short-TR/TE and long-TR/TE imaging sequences are used. In other words, a decrease in T_1 increases the NMR signal and potentially its contrast enhancement, whereas the simultaneous decrease in T_2 decreases T_2 contrast resolution between tissues, and vice versa. Under these conditions it will be very important to select an imaging method that emphasizes T_1, not T_2, in the final image. Conversely, because we have opposing influences on the image, it is unfortunately possible to pick an imaging method that includes both T_1 and T_2 and completely obscures tissue contrast differences.

GRAY SCALE AND CONTRAST AGENTS

The use of MRI contrast agents is based on the attempt to influence tissue relaxation parameters (T_1 and T_2). Certain substances enhance tissue relaxation because they can be induced by an external magnetic field to produce an additive magnetic field by a process of magnetic susceptibility. The ratio of induced magnetization to that of the external magnetic field is termed the *magnetic susceptibility* of the substance. Paramagnetic contrast agents have positive magnetic susceptibilities because their induced magnetic fields are additive to that of the applied magnetic field. A compound that has negative magnetic susceptibility is termed a *diamagnetic agent.* Positive magnetic susceptibility causes increased magnetic flux in the vicinity of the compound and thus produces increased relaxation in the surrounding tissue. Paramagnetic substances have magnetic moments only in the presence of an external magnetic field.

Ferromagnetism is characterized by established domains of magnetism that persist after the external magnetic field has been removed. Superparamagnetic agents have susceptibilities greater than those of paramagnetic agents, and unlike ferromagnetic substances, superparamagnetic substances lose their susceptibility in the absence of an external field. Paramagnetic susceptibility increases directly with external field strength, whereas both ferromagnetic and supermagnetic agents reach a point of saturation.

For paramagnetic agents, the magnitude of relaxation enhancement depends on the proximity of the paramagnetic agent to the nuclear spin. Paramagnetic agents are capable of realigning the bulk magnetic moment and therefore increasing T_1 relaxation rates. They also produce local magnetic inhomogeneities and thus shorten T_2 relaxation times as well.

Supermagnetic agents are particulates that have a greater induced magnetic moment than paramagnetic solutes, but are fixed and undergo less molecular tumbling. They thus create greater field heterogeneity and cause more T_2 shortening effects than T_1 shortening effects. For similar reasons, ferromagnetic-agent relaxation primarily affects T_2-weighted images.

The paramagnetic agents that have received the most attention are the paramagnetic lanthanide complexes, transition metals, and organic free radicals. In the lanthanide series, gadolinium and europium have the highest spin quantum numbers, and in the transition-metal group, Mn^{2+}, CR^{3+}, and Fe^{3+} are the most potent relaxation agents. Because of toxicity, both the lathanides and transition metals have been complexed with chelates; gadolinium has been complexed as Gd-DTPA, and manganese has been chelated as Mn-DTPA. Iron-containing compounds, such as Geritol and other drugs that contain ferrous or ferric salts, have been used as gastrointestinal enhancement agents. Parenteral iron has been administered as ferric hydroxamates and magnetite particulate compounds (Fe_3O_4). Iron has also been chelated with iron phenolates, such as Fe-HBED. Of the organic free radicals, nitroxides have been used in animal studies, but no clinical studies have been performed to date. In addition, nitroxide compounds are weak relaxation agents compared with some of the metal ions.

Particulate agents have been used mainly because they are phagocytosed by the reticuloendothelial system. Superparamagnetic or ferromagnetic particulates produce marked reductions in signal intensity in reticuloendothelial tissues in which they are concentrated. Again, this results from greater T_2 shortening than occurs with corresponding soluble paramagnetics. These agents have been used in the liver as "liver erasers" because they markedly reduce signal from normal liver tissue and produce increased conspicuity for any area of the liver not containing reticuloendothelial tissue (i.e., neoplastic metastases, etc.). Long-term retention by the reticuloendothelial system is a concern that is being addressed for these agents.

The use of contrast agents significantly changes tissue relaxation times and therefore the appearance of tissues on the MR image. Uncommonly, naturally occurring paramagnetic agents such as ^{17}O can change tissue contrast. Hemoglobin in blood clots can help to date hemorrhages as the iron passes from an oxygenated state to deoxygenated state and finally becomes hemosiderin in macrophages. Naturally occurring iron deposits in nuclei in the brain help to define the red nucleus, dentate nucleus, etc. Abnormal deposits in organs such as the liver in patients with hemochromatosis can significantly alter the image gray scale and thus the interpretation of the imaging data. Iron deposition in degenerative neurological disorders can be an indication of the underlying diagnosis. For example, in Huntington's chorea, increased iron is deposited in the caudate nucleus and putamen, whereas iron is deposited in the cerebral cortex in Alzheimer's disease and the posterior lateral putamen in Parkinson's disease.

Chapter 6

Clinical Applications of MRI

NEUROLOGICAL MRI

MRI has become the diagnostic modality of choice for evaluation of neurological diseases of the brain and spinal cord. Certain patients on life-support systems and with unstable physiological conditions still are more appropriately evaluated with CT or ultrasound. However, with a few exceptions (which would include ferromagnetic clips placed on aneurysms or the retina, or lesions in which detection of calcium is critical), study of the brain and spinal cord clearly is best performed using MRI.

MRI is excellent for evaluating primary and metastatic lesions of the central nervous system and for evaluating post-treatment courses (Figs. 6.1–6.6). Improvements in contrast-to-noise ratios and signal-to-noise ratios have led to excellent spatial resolution as well (Fig. 6.5). The ability to use MRI to characterize edema, primary tumor mass, and hemorrhage, resulting either from the cancer or from surgical or medical intervention, has been invaluable in assessing patients with neurological conditions (Figs. 6.2 and 6.4). MRI of infectious diseases and the consequences of infectious disease is providing new types of information often not obtainable with CT scanning alone (Figs. 6.7 and 6.8). MRI provides unique information regarding the consequences of intrathecal chemotherapy (Fig. 6.9). Common, as well as uncommon, afflictions of the central nervous system are more

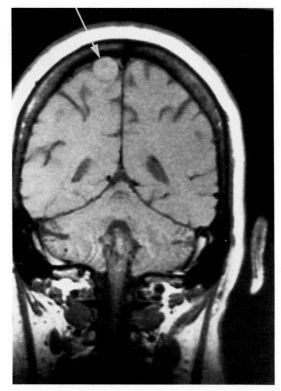

A

FIG. 6.1. Coronal (**A**, 800/20) and two axial (**B&C**, 2,000/20/80) MR images from a patient with a parasagittal parietal meningioma (*arrow*). The meningioma yields an intermediate signal on the T_1-weighted image (**A**) and increased signal intensity on the balanced MR image (**B**) and appears mottled on a heavily T_2-weighted image (**C**).

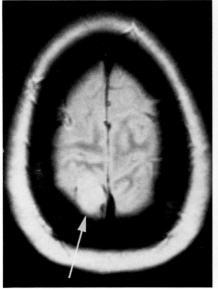

B

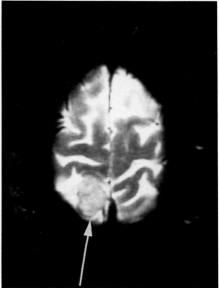

C

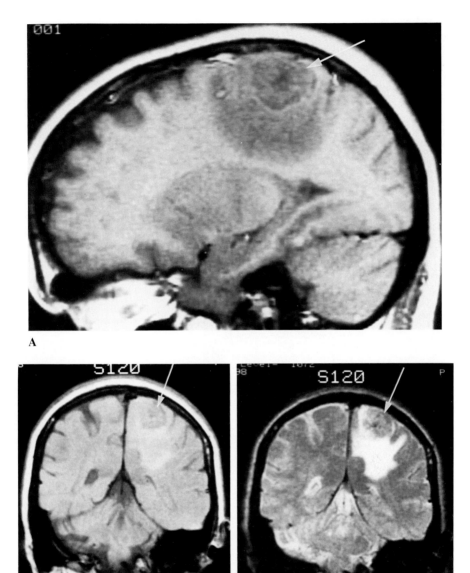

FIG. 6.2. Sagittal (**A,** 800/20) and coronal (**B&C,** 1,500/20/80) MR images form a 62-year-old woman with a well-circumscribed metastasis to the left parietal lobe (*arrow*). The primary tumor mass is surrounded by vasogenic edema following the white-matter distribution in the vicinity in the tumor and is seen as a low-intensity signal on the sagittal image, but a high-intensity signal on the most T_2-weighted image (**C**). The low-intensity 2–3-mm focus within the center of the tumor seen on the coronal T_2-weighted image (**C**) is a small area of hemorrhage containing hemosiderin. There was no calcium seen in this area on CT scanning. Vasogenic edema surrounding a metastasis is characteristic of primary and metastatic brain tumors and differs from the edema associated with infarction, which involves both gray and white matter (cellular edema).

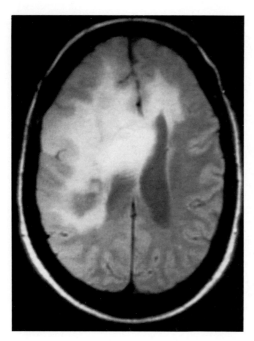

FIG. 6.3. Axial MR image at the level of the lateral ventricles (2,000/20) from a 48-year-old woman with an astrocytoma involving the right pons and right cerebral hemisphere, with invasion into the left hemisphere via the corpus callosum. This primary-brain-tumor-associated edema and mass effect are well seen following a white-matter distribution, nearly completely compressing the right lateral ventricle. There is some paraventricular edema progressing posteriorly, just lateral to the left lateral ventricle.

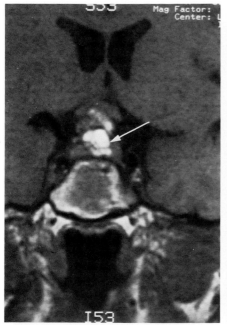

A

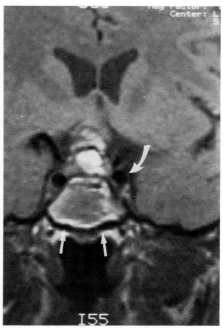

B

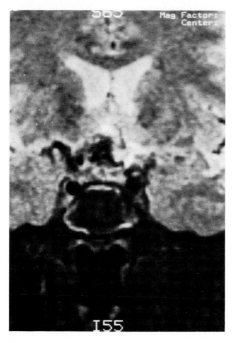

C

FIG. 6.4. Three coronal MRI studies (**A**, 800/20; **B**, 2,000/20; **C**, 2,000/80) through the pituitary in a 58-year-old man, previously diagnosed as having pituitary adenoma, postoperative at the time of imaging, who has had the sphenoid sinus packed with fat. The pituitary tumor (*long straight arrow*) had invaded the sphenoid sinus (*short white arrows*) and also invaded the suprasella cistern and hypothalamus. The sphenoid sinus has been packed with fat and shows a lower-intensity signal than normal fat because of revascularization. The surrounding white (or high-intensity) signal in all three images indicates circumferential hemorrhage around the fat contained with the sphenoid sinus. The tumor itself has areas of intermediate and old hemorrhage, as evidenced by high-intensity signal on the T_1 and balanced images (**A&B**). The low-intensity signal from the area on the T_2-weighted image (**C**) is due to hemosiderin and blood vessels capping the lesion in this area. The carotid arteries are well seen as flow voids within the cavernous sinus in this patient (*curved white arrow*).

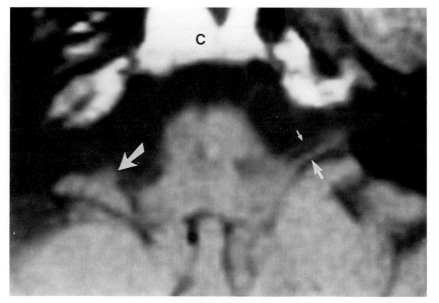

A

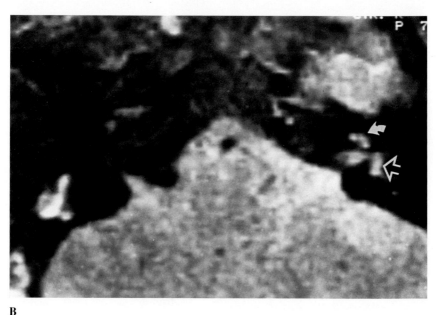

B

FIG. 6.5. The excellent spatial resolution of MRI is illustrated in this 65-year-old man with an incidental neuroma of the right facial nerve (*angled arrow*). The two axial images (**A&B,** 600/20 and 2,000/80) well reveal the normal anatomy of the normal left seventh (*small white arrow*) and eighth (*large white arrow*) cranial nerves in the more T₁-weighted image (**A**). The high-intensity structure (**C,** anteriorly) is bone marrow contained within the clivus and petrous ridges on either side. In the T₂-weighted image (**B**), normal CSF intensity is seen within the normal left internal auditory canal. On either side of this are seen the normal vestibular apparatus (*open arrow*) and cochlea (*curved white arrow*). The right seventh and eighth cranial nerves have been depressed slightly (**A**) because of the right facial neuroma arising from the superior aspect of the right facial nerve.

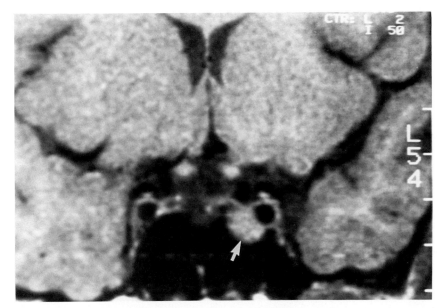

A

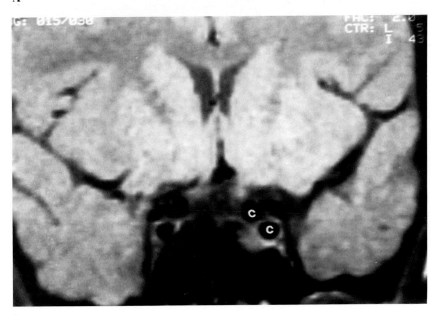

B

FIG. 6.6. Three axial images from a 24-year-old woman with a recurrent adenoma of the left cavernous sinus (*arrow*). The carotid siphon (**C**) in the cavernous sinus and the internal cerebral veins of the septum pellucidum (*small black arrows*) are well defined in this sequence. In the balanced, mostly proton-density image (**B**), the gray matter shows the highest signal intensity, followed by the white matter. The CSF in the lateral ventricles, which should have the highest proton density and therefore the highest-intensity (whitest) signal, is dark because of CSF flow and phase dispersion. The paired structures around the lateral ventricles represent the caudate nucleus (gray matter), internal capsule (white matter), and lentiform nucleus (gray matter). The adenoma has intermediate intensity on all three of these images (**A**, 800/25; **B&C**, 2,000/25/75).

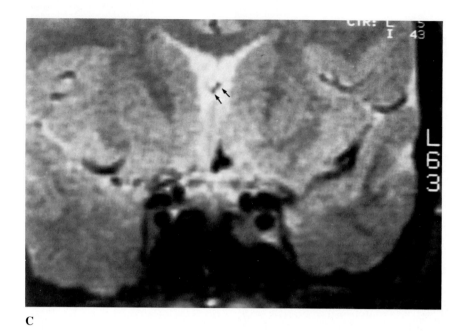

C

FIG. 6.6. continued.

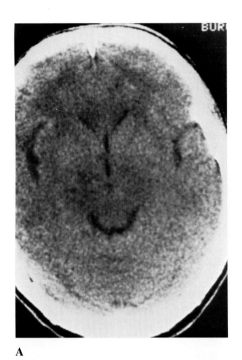

A

FIG. 6.7. Axial CT (**A**) and MRI (**B&C**, 2,000/40/80) from a patient with AIDS and a clinical question of neurological involvement. The patient was found to have progressive multifocal leukoencephalopathy that was not clearly seen on the CT scan, but was obvious at MRI evaluation. The abnormalities within the white matter are best seen on the balanced (**B**) MRI study, and the difference between this and the T_2-weighted gray-scale intensity is best seen in the occipital horns (*small white arrows*).

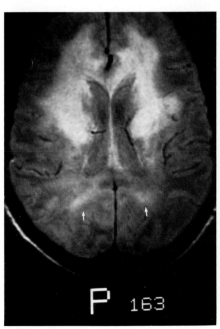

B

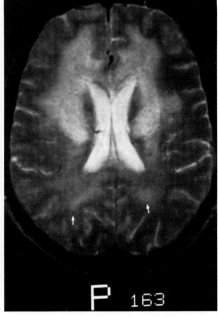

C

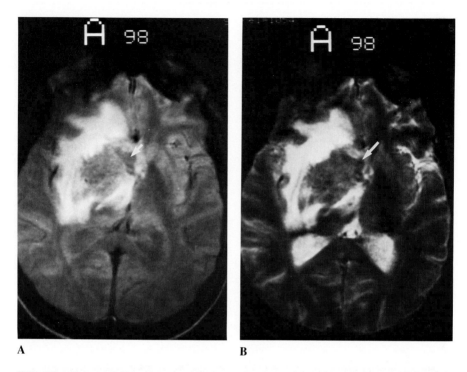

A   **B**

FIG. 6.8.   Two axial MRI studies in another patient with AIDS who had developed neurological lymphoma (*arrow*). Note the surrounding vasogenic, edema of white-matter (long T_2, brought out with long-TR/TE sequences) in this patient. The high-intensity posterior signal on the more T_2-weighted image (**B**) (**A, B;** 2,000/40/80) is due to CSF in the occipital horns of the ventricles.

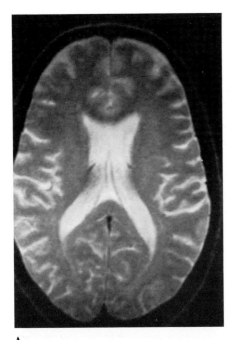

FIG. 6.9. These three axial MRI studies from a patient treated with intrathecal methotrexate document the development of methotrexate leukoencephalopathy. The three scans were obtained June 17, October 4, and December 3, 1985 (**A–C,** respectively). Only minimal increased signal intensity is seen within the paraventricular white matter on the study of June 17; however, on the study of October 4 there is noticeable increased signal intensity throughout the white matter (*white arrows*). At that time, a shunt had been placed in the right lateral ventricle (*black arrow*). By December 3, significant high-intensity abnormalities, due to the leukoencephalitis and edema, have developed throughout the white matter at the level of the lateral ventricles (**C**).

A

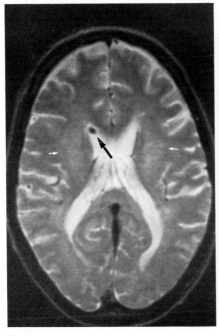

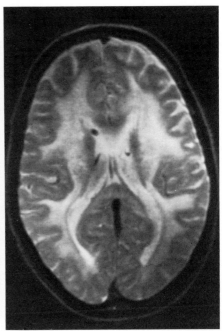

B   C

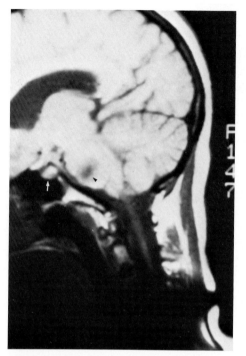

FIG. 6.10. Sagittal (**A,** 600/40) and axial (**B&C,** 1,500/40/80) MRI studies from a 34-year-old woman with sarcoidosis involving the pituitary (*small white arrow,* **A**), pons, and left temporal lobe (*large black arrows*). Although the lesion in the brainstem is obvious on all three images, the temporal lobe involvement is best defined on the T$_2$-weighted image (**C**). Note (**C**) the normal CSF in the internal auditory canal and left vestibular apparatus (*white arrows*). Also note the normal carotid arteries and basilar artery (*small black arrows,* **B**).

A

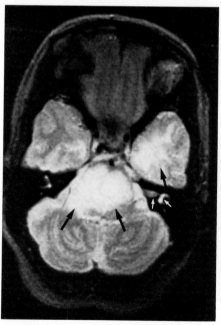

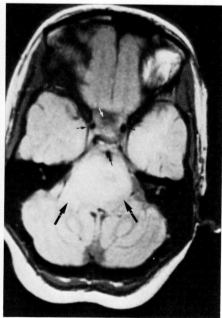

B   C

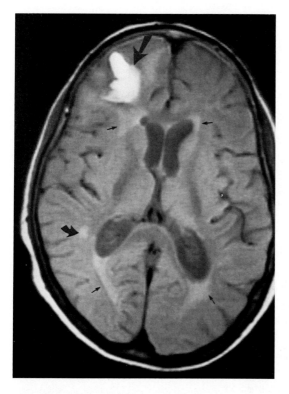

FIG. 6.11. Axial MR image (2,000/40) from a 75-year-old woman with amyloid angiopathy (congophillic angiopathy). This image, taken together with the CT findings (not shown) before and after intravenous administration of contrast material, illustrates the complimentary nature of CT and MRI for evaluating some neurological conditions. In this case, the findings of a recent frontal hematoma (*black angled arrow*) with multiple white-matter UBOs (unidentified bright objects), one of the largest of which is marked (*curved black arrow,* although there are many others in the juxtacortical area), suggest long-standing and recurrent infarction with an acute right frontal bleed (*large black arrow*). The differential diagnosis in this case would include an acute bleed (or a bleed into an infarct or an acute bleed into a tumor). Bleeding into a tumor is less frequent; in addition, the increased density on pre- and post-contrast CT studies was suggestive of a hematoma rather than a bleed into a tumor. In addition, the high density was peripheral on sagittal MR images, and bleeding into a tumor often is more centrally located. A third differential point in this case will be follow-up evaluation over time. With MRI, the hematoma will show central increased intensity on partial-saturation sequences over time, as hemoglobin is converted to deoxyhemoglobin. The clinical history in this case was about 1 week in duration. Also note some paraventricular high-intensity signal (*small black arrows*), probably due to edema.

easily detected and managed using the excellent diagnostic capabilities of MRI (Figs. 6.10 and 6.11).

MRI of the Vertebral Column

MRI of the vertebral column is rapidly replacing more conventional approaches such as CT. MRI has all but replaced myelography. One of the advances that has made this expansion of MRI possible is the elimination of CSF flow artifacts. Techniques involving CSF flow compensation in spin-echo imaging, combined with gradient refocusing, have considerably improved image resolution for the spinal cord and its surrounding contents. The gains in imaging quality made possible by eliminating flow- and phase-encoding-related artifacts are indicated in Fig. 6.12. The spatial resolution and contrast resolution achieved using the techniques of CSF-

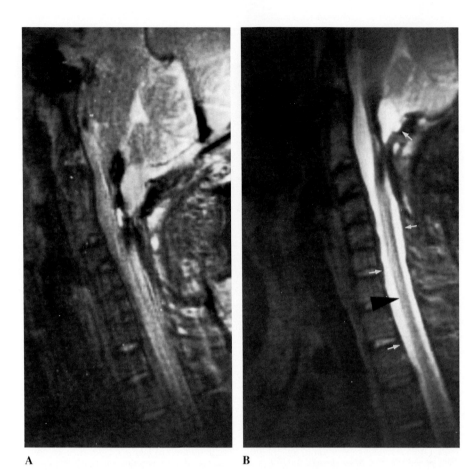

A   **B**

FIG. 6.12. Comparison of conventional T_2-weighted spin-echo image of the cervical spine with one obtained using CSF-flow-compensation methods in a patient with a postoperative spinal cord glioma. **A**: Conventional spin-echo image (TR = 2,000 msec, TE = 80 msec). **B**: CSF-flow-compensated spin-echo image using CSF-gated acquisition and gradient rephasing, with an effective TR of approximately 2,200 msec (gated to every third heart beat) and fourth echo at TE = 80 msec (study performed approximately 9 months after **A**). On the conventional image (**A**), CSF oscillatory motion causes reduced CSF signal intensity (signal loss) and spatial mismapping of this signal (phase-shift images), seen as vertical stripes across the whole image. These reduce image quality by partially obscuring the spinal cord and reducing the contrast of the CSF/thecal sac and CSF/spinal cord interfaces. On the CSF-flow-compensated image (**B**), CSF-flow artifacts have been almost completely eliminated, improving visualization of the spinal cord and extradural structures. Focal regions of decreased signal intensity within the cord represent magnetic-susceptibility effects, likely secondary to hemosiderin deposits. The focal region of increased signal intensity posterior below the foramen magnum on both images corresponds to a resolving cystic collection, possibly containing old blood. CSF gating was performed using a peripheral detector attached to a fingertip that detects capillary perfusion (courtesy of J. Rubin and A. Wright). Using gating in the spine and head to improve image quality does not increase acquisition time. Gradient rephasing was performed using an echo train of TE = 20, 40, 60, and 80 msec, which provides velocity compensation on even echoes. Similar results would be obtained using a flow-compensated pulse sequence incorporating additional gradient pulses to rephase flowing protons. CSF gating and gradient rephasing eliminate flow artifacts arising from different mechanisms and so are synergistic. Implementation of these techniques, particularly on T_2-weighted images of the spine or head, permits improved image quality without increasing imaging time (CSF on gated image, *white arrow;* cervical spinal cord, *black arrowhead*). (Courtesy of J. B. Rubin, Stanford University.)

flow-compensated spin-echo imaging and gradient-echo rephasing are truly remarkable and are possible without the use of intrathecal contrast agents.

Another approach to the elimination of flow-related artifacts is indicated in Fig. 6.13. Techniques of flow imaging—in this case, steady-state refocusing and gradient-recalled echoes (SSRGR)—allow NMR images to be obtained that reflect only moving protons (or flowing protons) in the scanning aperture. Considerable improvement in image resolution of the cervical spinal cord is afforded because the moving CSF is shown as a high-intensity signal around it, whereas the more conventional spin-echo images can be quite confusing.

Because of the reduced oscillatory pulsations, there has been less difficulty with CSF-flow-related artifacts in the lower lumbar spine. In addition, often there is considerable extradural fat that affords a defined interface between the dura and its intradural contents and the bony spinal canal and its surrounding contents. By obtaining spin-echo images, a so-called matrisimide effect can be achieved by displaying the surrounding fat as a low-intensity signal, whereas the relatively stationary CSF is seen as a signal of very high intensity (Fig. 6.14). The major problem in MRI examination of the lumbar spine has been that orthogonal planes to the intervertebral disc spaces have not been available until fairly recently. However, with the development of the capability to reconstruct MRI data along the plane of the intervertebral discs, considerable progress has been made in MRI diagnostic capabilities in disc disease (Fig. 6.15).

These advances, combined with the intrinsic ability of MRI to reveal the bone marrow within the vertebrae of the vertebral column, have led to exquisite diagnostic capability with regard to primary abnormalities of the bony vertebral column (Fig. 6.16). These techniques have enabled MRI to make significant contributions in nearly every classification of pathological process involving the vertebral column, its contents, and surrounding tissues. MRI is the modality of choice for evaluating congenital abnormalities of the cord itself (Figs. 6.17 and 6.18) and acquired abnormalities such as primary cord neoplasms.

MRI is also the imaging modality of choice for evaluating postoperative patients. Residual deformity, either due to the surgery or not corrected by the surgery, can be accurately evaluated, as shown in the case of the residual postoperative cyst in Fig. 6.19. Flow imaging can also define the dynamic consequences of the surgical procedure in terms of functional stenosis and lack of CSF flow. Laterally placed disc fragments and stenosis of the foramina are similarly well delineated by this process, and it now appears possible, in many cases, to distinguish residual fibrosis from recurrent disc disease (Figs. 6.20–6.23).

MRI of the Thorax

Many of the techniques that have been developed in MRI of the brain and vertebral column have found application for examination of the thorax. Specifically troublesome in this area has been the control of both respiratory motion and cardiovascular motion. These excursions cause the same phase-encoded and flow artifacts seen in imaging of the vertebral column and brain and have been, to some extent,

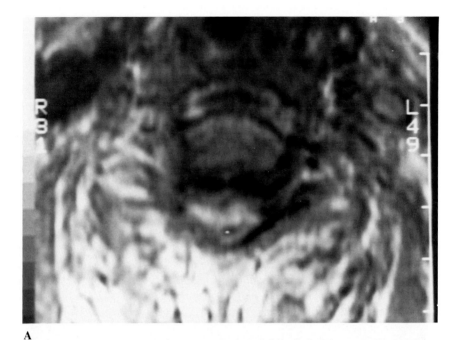

A

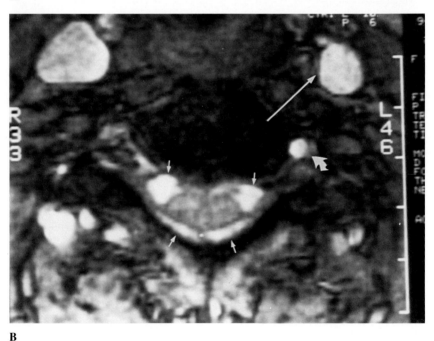

B

FIG. 6.13. Conventional spin-echo (**A**) and flow imaging (**B,** SSRGR method) illustrating the advantages of flow imaging and static-tissue suppression in evaluating the cervical cord. Because of phase encoding and CSF-flow artifacts, the conventional spin-echo image has little diagnostic value. However, and MR image obtained to illustrate flow phenomena indicates the cervical cord surrounded by CSF (*short white arrows*). Other types of information are now available as well, including good anatomic visualization of the vertebral arteries (*curved arrow), jugular vein (long arrow*), and other venous structures in the posterior neck.

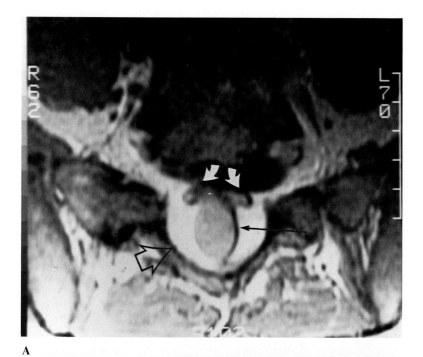

A

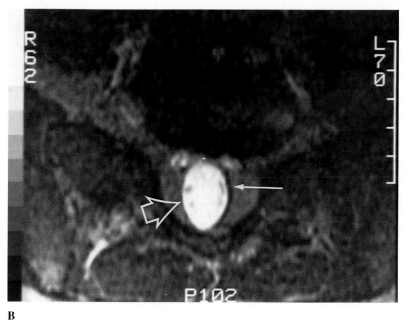

B

FIG. 6.14. First-echo (**A**) and second-echo (**B**) (2,500/40/80) normal MR images of the lumbar spine. The imaging sequence, combined with the extradural fat (*open black arrow*) and white CSF produced on the second echo (*open white arrow*), provides excellent detail of the dura and the exiting nerve roots (*curved white arrows*). Also shown is the chemical-shift effect to the right of the dural sack (*long black and white arrows*). These images were obtained without flow compensation, as the CSF pulsations in the lumbar spine are relatively small, and the extradural fat provides excellent surrounding contrast.

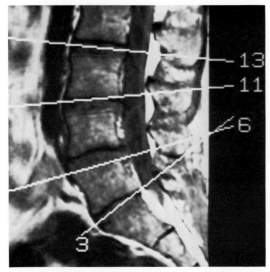

A

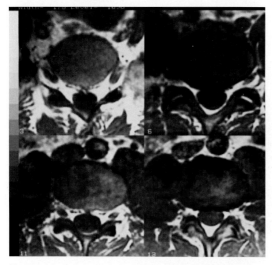

B

FIG. 6.15. Sagittal (**A**) and axial oblique images of the normal lumbar spine. The numbers on the sagittal image correspond to the axial images obtained at that level. The ability to obtain MR images orthogonal to the intervertebral discs has greatly improved MRI capability in diagnosing disc disease. (Courtesy of the General Electric Co.)

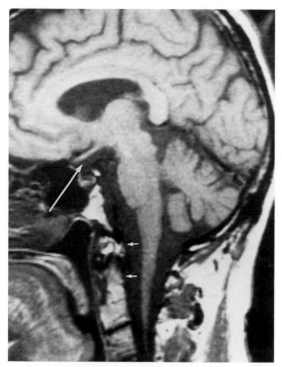

A

FIG. 6.16. Two MR images from a spin-echo sequence illustration extensive destruction of the first and second cervical vertebrae in a patient with rheumatoid arthritis (*small arrows*). One of the optic nerves is well shown in this sequence (*long arrow*), as is the pituitary gland (*curved arrow*). The mesencephalon (1), pons (2), splenium of the corpus callosum (3), and cerebellum (4) are marked. Note the fourth ventricle just before the number 4 and the black flow void of the internal cerebral vein anterior to the splenium, (the vein of Galen inferior and posterior to the splenium, and the straight sinus descending posterior to the splenium and above the cerebellum. The straight sinus joins the superior sagittal sinus in the torcular (t).

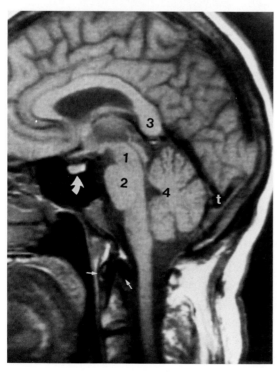

B

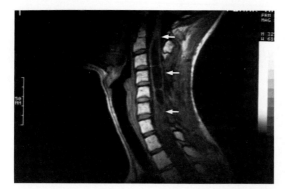

FIG. 6.17. Syringomyelia of the upper cervical cord is well shown on this T₁-weighted image, indicated by the low signal emanating from the cystic syrinx (*white arrows*). Note the relatively high signal emanating from the subcutaneous fat and fatty marrow within the vertebral bodies anteriorly (0.3-T permanent magnet; 388/16). (Courtesy of Fonar Inc.)

FIG. 6.18. Sagittal (**A**) and two axial (**B&C**) T₁-weighted MR images from a patient with diastematomyelia indicating a syringomyelia of the upper lumbar and lower thoracic spinal cord (*black arrows*), the split cord on an axial image (*long arrow*), and an associated horse-shoe kidney (*curved arrows*). Note the flow void of the entire inferior vena cava; the kidney can be seen lying anterior to the cava (**A**).

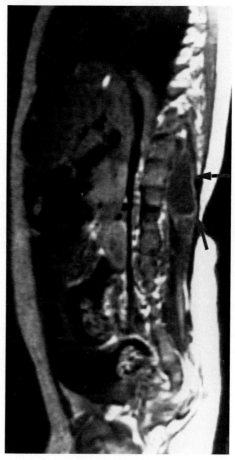

A

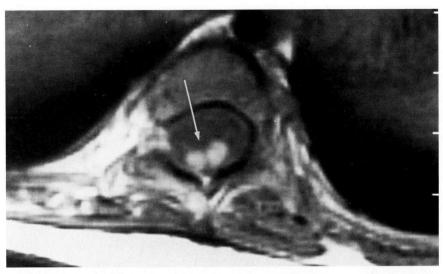

B

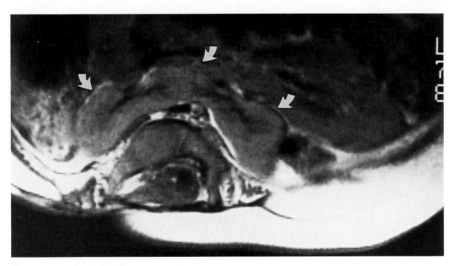

C

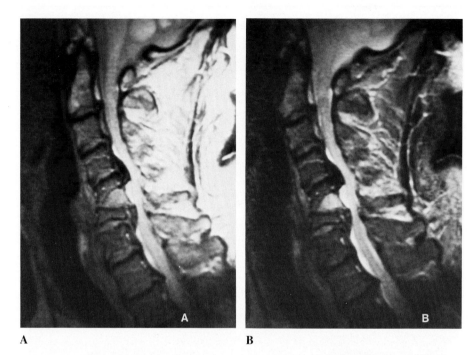

A   B

FIG. 6.19. MRI study from a patient who has had a dorsal cervical laminectomy for degenerative cervical spine disease. This sequence includes a four-echo spin-echo sequence (**A–D**) and a low-flip-angle/gradient-recalled-echo sequence (**E**). The spin-echo sequence has been gated; so there is little phase-encoded or CSF-flow artifact. Note the anterior cyst (*curved solid white arrow*) and a severe impression from postoperative fibrosis above it (*open partial arrow*).

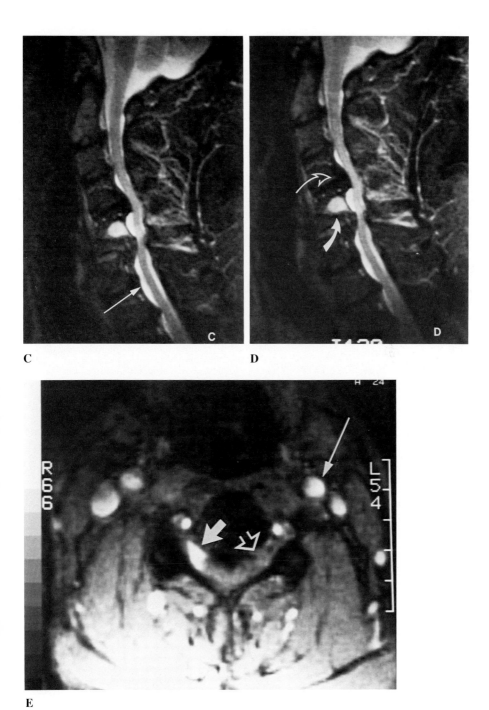

C   D

E

FIG. 6.19. (*continued*). Also note the increasing signal intensity for CSF and decreasing relative signal intensity for the spinal cord and lower cerebellum (**C** *long white arrow* is CSF). Flow is indicated by high-intensity signal (**E**), indicating that there is no CSF flow along the left side (*open arrowhead*) as opposed to the right side (*arrowhead*). The vertebral arteries are seen anterolaterally above these two arrowheads, as are the carotid artery and jugular veins (**E,** *long arrow*). (TR = 400 msec; SE 25/50/75/100; 30° tip angle; 22/12).

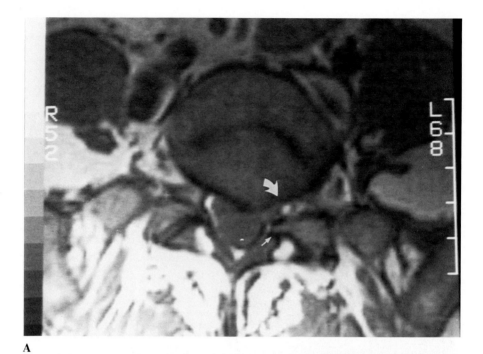

A

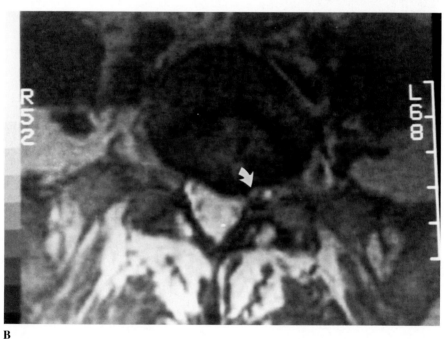

B

FIG. 6.20. T$_1$-weighted (**A**) and T$_2$-weighted (**B**) images of the lumbar spine in a patient with lateral-recess compression on the left. The abnormality is produced by an eccentric lateral bulge of the disc and also hypertrophy of the facet at this level. The abnormality is indicated by a lack of extradural fat (*curved arrow*) on the T$_1$-weighted image and a lack of CSF in the lateral recess on the T$_2$-weighted image (*curved arrow*). (abnormal facet, *short white arrow*). Compare with Fig. 6.14.

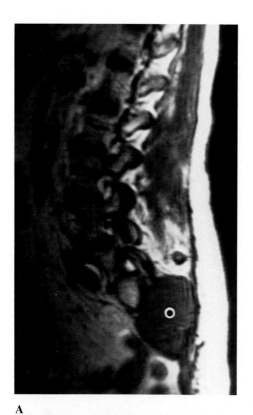

A

FIG. 6.21. Sagittal (**A**) and axial (**B**) MR images from a patient with a sacral chordoma (*bullet*). The chordoma is well defined and is shown to have invaded the bone on this partial-saturation sequence (TR = 800 msec; TE = 20 msec).

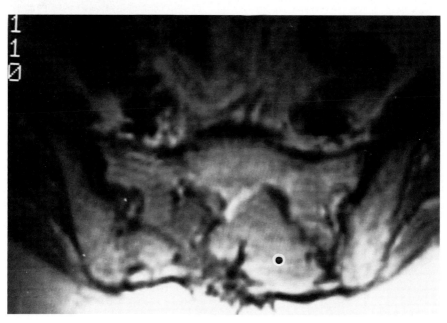

B

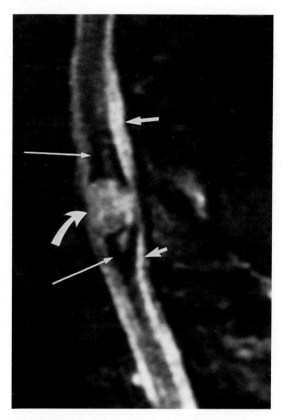

FIG. 6.22. A heavily T$_2$-weighted MR image from a patient with a primary tumor of the spinal cord. Note that the tumor (*curved arrow*) is surrounded by hemosiderin (*long arrows*), and both of these components are well defined by the CSF of relatively high signal (*short arrows*). The patient also had atrophy of the cord below this level that is not well shown in this image. The imaging sequence reveals very little soft-tissue definition, because muscle, fat, and fatty marrow have large molecules tumbling at very slow speeds, resulting in short T$_2$ relaxation times, having undergone nearly complete T$_2$ relaxation. Hemosiderin appears black because of the marked T$_2$ relaxation produced by the hemosiderin (see Chapter 5). CSF appears white because the small salt molecules in CSF are tumbling much more rapidly than the resonant frequency of the protons at 1.5 T, and therefore little T$_2$ relaxation occurs. T$_2$ for the cancer is long because of the edema and large amount of extracellular/intracellular fluid present in most tumors. There may also be slow flow enhancement and more recent areas of hemorrhage, accounting for the mottled texture of the cancer's image.

corrected by similar techniques. MRI has been found to be an excellent modality for elucidating the normal anatomy of the thorax (Figs. 6.24–6.27). Vascular structures have been differentiated from other solid tissues by taking advantage of the flow void yielded by rapidly flowing blood and using narrow-flip-angle gradient-recalled echo techniques to produce a high-intensity signal from flowing blood. This feature of MRI has been useful for evaluating patients suspected of having dissection, as in Fig. 6.28, and for follow-up evaluation of shunt patency, as in Fig. 6.29. Gating has also been useful for examination of the heart itself without the use of narrow tip angles and gradient-recalled echoes (Fig. 6.30).

Irradiated bone marrow undergoes fatty replacement after some period of time, and the invasion of this high-intensity fat signal on T$_1$-weighted images has been useful in diagnosing metastases and neoplastic recurrence (Fig. 6.31). Motion has been a problem to some extent in evaluating patients with mediastinal masses, but applications of MRI of the thorax are progressing steadily, and MRI is being used more and more in evaluating intrathoracic abnormalities (Fig. 6.32).

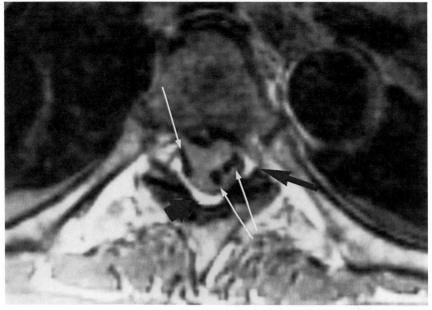

A

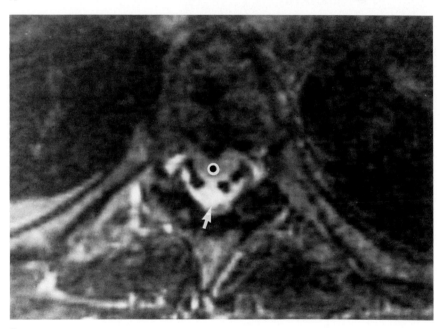

B

FIG. 6.23. This MRI sequence was obtained from a patient with vague symptoms involving the lower extremities and pain in the middle and upper back. A T$_1$-weighted partial-saturation study (**A**), a T$_2$-weighted spin-echo sequence (**B**), and a narrow-tip-angle/gradient-recalled-echo sequence (**C**) were obtained from this patient.

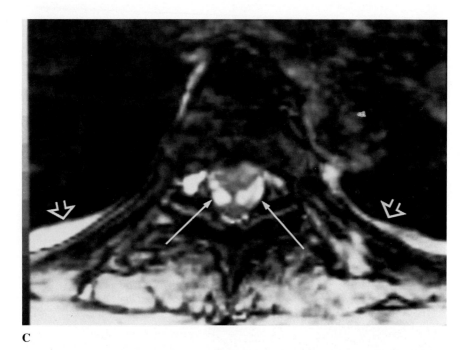

C

FIG. 6.23. (*continued*). The MRI study reveals that the patient had an AV malformation (AVM) of the thoracic spinal cord (*long white arrows*). In the partial-saturation image the extradural fat is seen (*black arrows*) outlining the dural sac, and the AVM is seen as a flow void within the dura (*long white arrows*). On the spin-echo sequence the relatively static CSF is seen as a high-intensity white signal (*white arrow*). The cord is seen surrounded by the CSF and the AVM (the cord is indicated by the black-and-white bullet). In the narrow-tip-angle/gradient-recalled-echo sequence, moving protons are seen as a high-intensity signal revealing the full extent of the AVM (*long white arrows*). The bilateral pleural effusions are best seen in the flow-weighted image as well, indicating that the effusion is freely flowing. It is this motion that explains the lack of signal that should have been seen from the effusions on the spin-echo (or T_2-weighted) image.

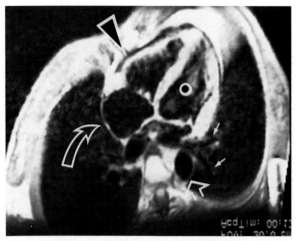

A

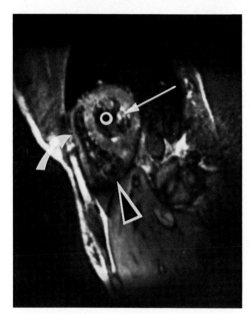

B

FIG. 6.24. Four-chamber long-axis (**A**) and short-axis (**B**) gated MR images from a normal volunteer. The examination was performed at 0.38 T on a resistive iron-core magnet using a standard spin-echo sequence, with the TR interval determined by the heart rate, and a TE of 15 msec. Oblique views and radial views around any point are available using this technique, and an interesting artifact occurs where radial planes intersect, creating a void that appears as a curved linear low density running through the image (Fig. 6.77). The normal anatomy seen in this view is as follows: left ventricle (*bullet*), right ventricle (*black-and-white arrowhead*), right atrium (*open white curved arrow*), left atrium (*open white arrowhead*). Small pulmonary veins are flowing into the left atrium (*small arrows*), and the main pulmonary artery just above the pulmonary valve is indicated (*curved white arrow*). This arrow is projecting outside of the patient, passing through an oblique view of the anterior chest wall. The black-and-white arrowhead's body is superimposed over the liver in this projection. Note the papillary muscle in the left ventricle (*long white arrow*). These views are the same projections commonly obtained during ultrasound examination of the heart. (Courtesy of Dr. F. Burbank.)

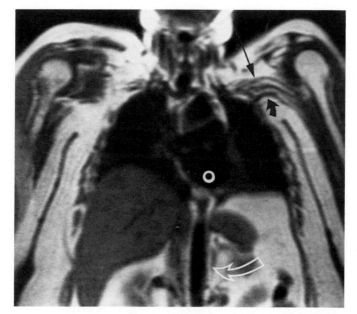

A

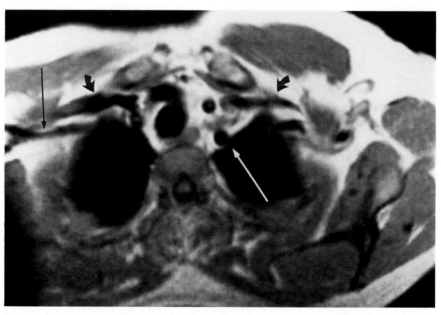

B

FIG. 6.25. Coronal (**A**) and axial (**B**) MR images of the thoracic inlet in a normal individual. The subclavian arteries (*long arrows*) and subclavian veins (*curved black arrows*) are well delineated from the surrounding mediastinal tissue and other soft tissues. Other vascular structures, such as the descending abdominal aorta (*open white arrow*) and left atrium (*bullet*), are also well defined.

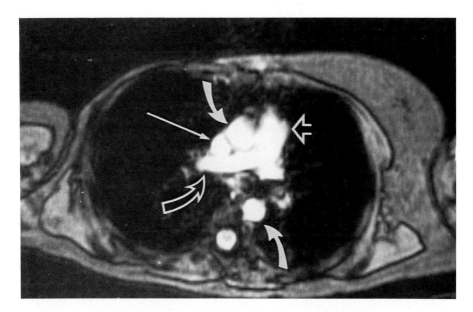

FIG. 6.26. Small-flip-angle/gradient-recalled-echo flow-weighted axial MR image at the level of the main pulmonary artery in a patient who has had right radical mastectomy for breast carcinoma. The flow-weighted image reveals excellent vascular detail, with a high-intensity signal from all flowing blood. CSF also shows high intensity in this image because of CSF pulsations. Also shown are main pulmonary artery (*open arrowhead*), aortic root and descending thoracic aorta (*curved solid arrows*), superior vena cava (*long arrow*), and right main pulmonary artery (*open curved arrow*). The high-intensity CSF signal is seen posterior and slightly medial to the descending thoracic aorta. Low-intensity signal coming from static tissues is markedly suppressed with this technique.

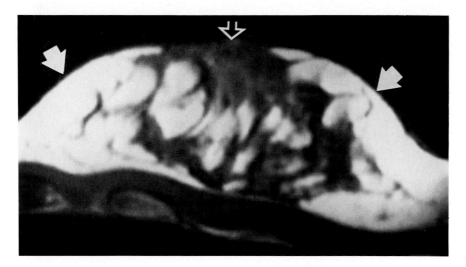

FIG. 6.27. Axial T$_1$-weighted MR image of a normal breast indicating the glandular breast tissue (*open white arrow*) and surrounding fat (*solid arrowheads*). The chest wall is seen posterior to the breast, and the dark structure inferior to this is the lung.

131

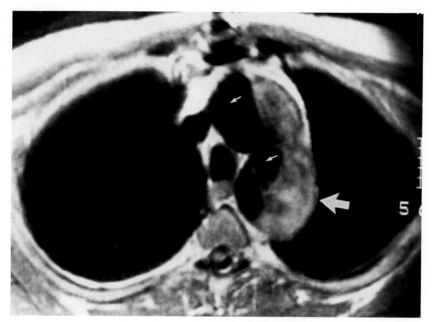

A

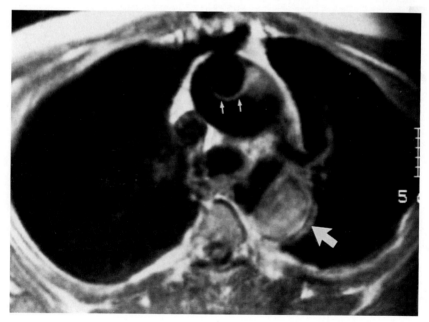

B

FIG. 6.28. Two axial MR images at the level of the middle and lower aortic arch in a patient with an aortic type-A dissection. The intimal flap is well defined against the flow void within the true channel (*small arrows*). The partially clotted false lumen is seen as a low-intensity gray signal (*large arrows*). Note the metallic artifacts from sternal wires anteriorly.

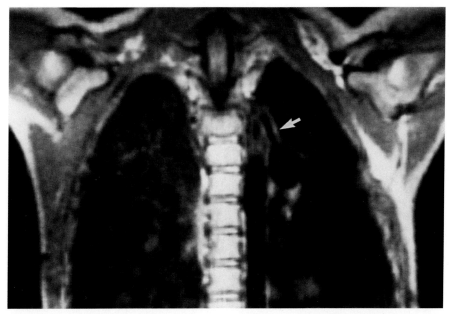

A

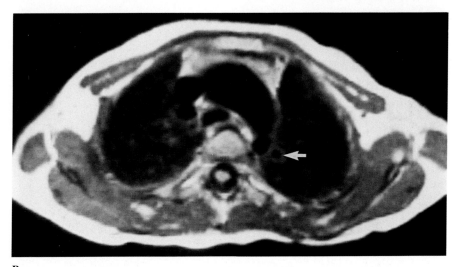

B

FIG. 6.29. Coronal (**A**) and axial (**B**) MR images from a patient with a previously placed gortex shunt between the left main pulmonary artery and the left subclavian artery (*arrow*). The black flow-void signal indicates that the shunt is patent.

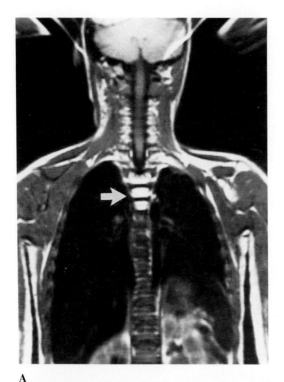

FIG. 6.30. Coronal MR image (**A**) and axial CT scan (**B**) from a patient successfully treated with radiation therapy for rhabdomyosarcoma and a sagittal (**C**) MR image from a patient with previous irradiation for lymphoma. The patient now presents with a positive bone scan and positive MR image of the 11th thoracic vertebra and recurrence of Hodgkin's disease in the bone marrow of the 11th thoracic vertebra. This series illustrates the normal occurrence of fatty marrow after irradiation and the difficulty in detecting this phenomenon with CT scanning (*arrows,* **A** & **B**). Recurrent Hodgkin's disease in the 11th thoracic vertebra (**C**) is indicated by the infiltration of fat within the T11 vertebral body, seen as a low-intensity signal (*arrow*) (TR = 800 msec, TE = 20 msec). The CT scan also reveals a small left pleural effusion, and Hickman catheter is present in the right anterior chest wall.

A

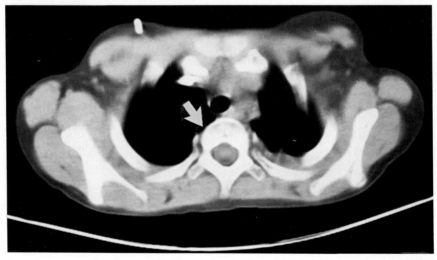

B

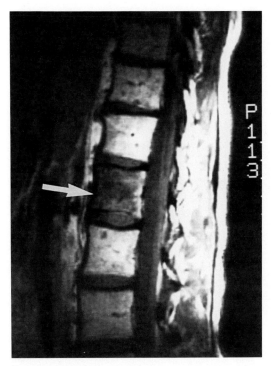

C

FIG. 6.30. continued.

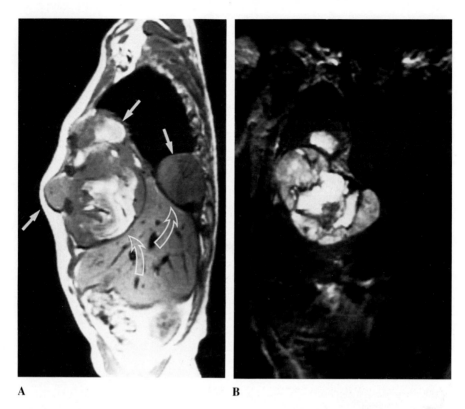

A **B**

FIG. 6.31. Sagittal MR image (**A,** TR = 800 msec, TE = 25 msec) and coronal more T$_2$-weighted MR image (**B,** TR = 2,000 msec, TE = 80 msec) from a patient with a malignant schwannoma of the thorax. The sagittal view reveals invasion of the anterior chest wall and a second focus posteriorly (*solid arrows*). There is also inversion of the hemidiaphragm and compression of the liver, both anteriorly and posteriorly (*open arrows*). The coronal view reveals the complexity of the tumor, with areas of calcification, edema, hemorrhage, and large blood vessels contained within it.

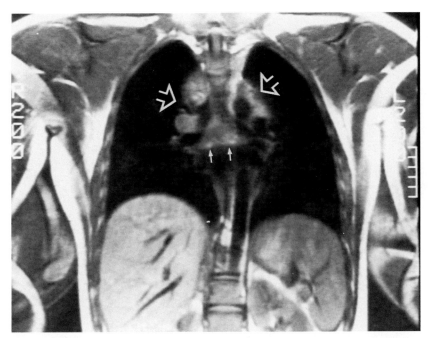

A

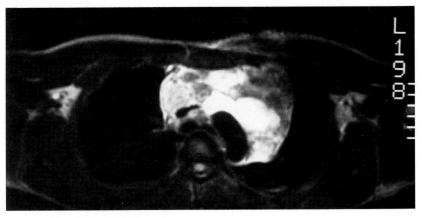

B

FIG. 6.32. A: Coronal MR image from a patient with mediastinal lymphoma. **B:** Axial MR image at the level of the aortic arch in a second patient with mediastinal lymphoma (heavily T$_2$-weighted, 2000/75).

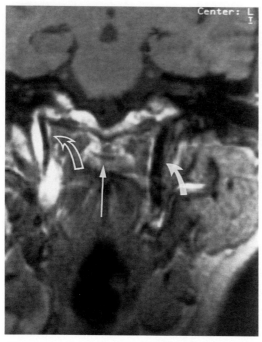

C

FIG. 6.32. (*continued*). **C:** Coronal MR image (same patient as in **A**) in which an incidental dissection of the right carotid artery is identified. The lymphoma (**A**) involves the right superior mediastinum, right hilum, left superior mediastinum overlapping the aorta and left main pulmonary artery (*open arrows*), and the subcarinal area (*small arrows*). The axial image reveals a common characteristic of mediastinal lymphoma in that there is an area of very high intensity within the lymphomatous mass on the image that is heavily T_2-weighted. The carotid dissection (*open arrow*) reveals hematoma to the right of the carotid artery. Part of the lumen is still patent (*signal void*). Compare with the normal left carotid (*solid curved arrow*). The high-intensity signal between the two carotids (*long white arrow*) represents fat in the clivus and dorsum sulla. Above that is seen CSF, and within that the basilar artery is seen in cross section as a flow void. Just to the left of the base of the curved solid white arrow is seen a normal parotid gland. Note the aliasing artifacts present on the right and left lateral aspects (**A**). These represent wraparound images of the upper arms.

MRI OF BLOOD

Motion Imaging with Magnetic Resonance

One important component of the information in NMR experiments is motion, or flow, and imaging of blood flow has now become a clinical reality. Attention first focused on flowing blood in MR images when blood vessels were imaged in axial sections and were variously seen as bright, dark, or intermediate structures. These effects were quickly associated with the velocity and direction of the flowing blood and the pulsing sequence used. Increased signal intensity was found to be related either to in-plane flow or flow-related brightness often seen in the first entry slice

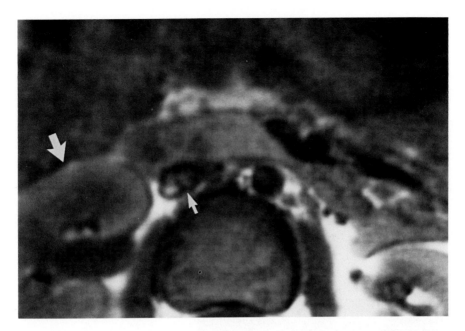

FIG. 6.33. Axial MR image at the level of the transverse duodenum indicating the entry-slice phenomenon (*small arrow*) in the inferior vena cava (the first slice in this sequence). No signal is obtained from the aorta. The duodenum is crossing anterior to the vena cava, and the right kidney is seen (*large arrow*). Flow-related phenomena, such as this entry-slice enhancement, are due to incoming protons that are completely relaxed and therefore provide a stronger signal than other protons that are only partially saturated. This (like even-echo rephasing) often creates some difficulty in interpretation, especially when the slice is perpendicular to the direction of flow.

of an imaging procedure (Figs. 6.33–6.35). This results from blood entering the imaging volume with full magnetization (as opposed to protons that have already experienced a 90° RF pulse and thus are capable of producing a brighter signal than stationary protons). Signal brightness is also caused by even-echo rephasing, which occurs on the even-echo images of a multiple spin-echo sequence. Each time protons are flipped 360° following an initial 90° pulse, complete rephasing of the protons results, and even echoes thus produce a higher-intensity signal than odd echoes (see Fig. 6.42). Decreased signal from within blood vessels usually results from either high velocity or turbulence. Protons passing quickly through the imaging volume do not receive a full 90° or 180° RF pulse, and turbulent flow causes phase dispersion and resultant loss of signal. Cross-sectional imaging of laminar flow has also been found to produce unusual target and ring configurations within blood vessels because of the same complex interaction between flowing blood and the characteristics of the pulsing sequence. Research has now moved away from incidental observations made during clinical cross-sectional imaging to efforts to acquire flow-related data to facilitate clinical management of patients. There are two broad categories of approaches to flow imaging: (1) time-of-flight effects, which

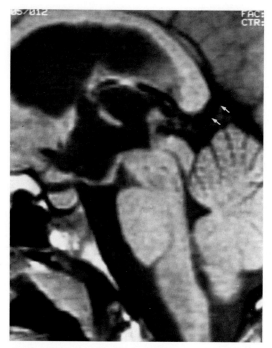

A

FIG. 6.34. Sagittal (**A**) and magnified sagittal (**B**) T$_1$-weighted MR images from a patient with an aneurysm of the great vein of Galen (*arrows*). The rapid flow in these abnormal vessels is seen as a signal void. Flow information is thus available using more or less conventional or standard MRI pulsing sequences.

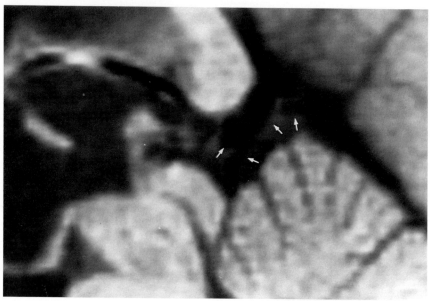

B

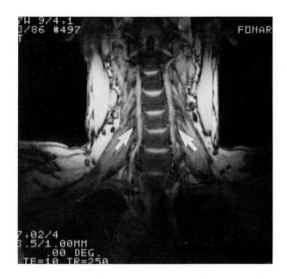

FIG. 6.35. A coronal T_1-weighted image obtained with a 0.3-T permanent magnet reveals that in-plane flow yields a high-intensity signal, in this case from the vertebral arteries (*arrows*). (Courtesy of Fonar Inc.)

depend on spin excitation history, and (2) flow-dependent or motion-dependent phase shifts, usually induced by bipolar gradients.

Time-of-Flight-Methods

MRI of blood flow has benefited considerably from previous efforts to increase patient throughput. Initial efforts in this regard included using higher magnetic field strengths (to improve signal-to-noise ratio) and pulsing sequences based on echo planar synthesis or conjugate synthesis in which half of the data are acquired in Fourier space and the other half are generated by software prior to the reconstruction, i.e., $N = 1/2$. More recently, efforts to shorten TR intervals, and thereby reduce imaging time, have resulted in the development of small flip angles and gradient-recalled echoes. This approach is now being used extensively in time-of-flight blood-flow imaging. The reduced-flip-angle/gradient-reversal techniques are able to shorten imaging times by twofold to fourfold, depending on the objective of the study. These time savings are achieved by using an RF pulse that is less than 90° (typically 20° to 60°), which allows shorter TR intervals. The spin-echo is produced using a gradient-recalled echo as opposed to an RF-induced spin-echo (Fig. 6.36). Blood, in contrast to its appearance on conventional MR images, yields a higher signal intensity relative to static tissue. The high intensity for flowing blood is caused by the continuous entry of unsaturated spins into the imaging slice. Thus, in rapidly flowing blood, a complete washout of saturated spins occurs, whereas the stationary spins for surrounding tissues are partially saturated when they experience the next RF pulse, leading to diminished signal intensity relative to that for the flowing blood. This type of pulsing sequence is very sensitive to spin density,

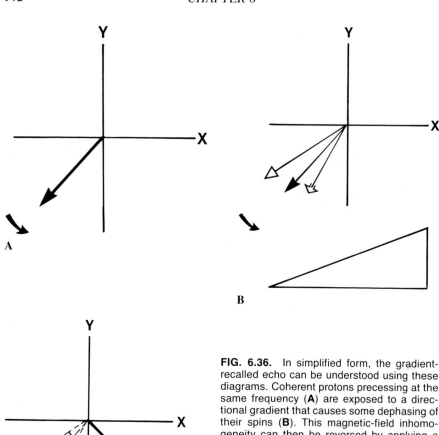

FIG. 6.36. In simplified form, the gradient-recalled echo can be understood using these diagrams. Coherent protons precessing at the same frequency (**A**) are exposed to a directional gradient that causes some dephasing of their spins (**B**). This magnetic-field inhomogeneity can then be reversed by applying a gradient in the opposite direction (**C**). Because the dephasing and rephasing are produced by magnetic forces in the gradient field, the information is directly related to T_2^*. The advantage is that the echo time can be considerably shorter than with a conventional spin-echo technique. The method is also useful for enhancing tissue magnetic susceptibility and therefore is useful for determining the age of a hemorrhage and for imaging with contrast agents.

and the high proton density of blood may be an additional factor contributing to the increased signal intensity. In addition, signal loss from phase-dispersion effects is decreased when the echo time is very short. And the echo itself is caused by the reversal of the readout gradient, which does not affect the signal phase of flowing blood.

Reduced-flip-angle/gradient-reversal techniques are also being used in other types of clinical evaluation (*vide infra*). Pathological conditions in which the tissue water content is increased provide high object contrast. Elevated water content is associated with increases in T_1, T_2, and nuclear density. In conventional spin-echo imaging with 90° flip angles, lengthening T_1 causes decreased signal intensity. Only at long TR values do T_2 and nuclear-density effects overshadow T_1 effects. However, using a reduced flip angle and values of TR that are less than T_1, signal intensity increases, peaks, and then decreases as the flip angle is reduced. Thus, this approach to MR imaging tends to reverse the dependence of signal intensity on T_1 effects. Another advantage that accrues from using gradient echoes (field echoes) concerns the problem posed by systemic absorption rates and power-deposition restrictions in high-field-strength imaging. Elimination of the need to use 90° and 180° RF pulses significantly reduces the deposited RF power.

A major concern in using partial-flip-angle MR imaging is that contrast drops rapidly as a function of flip angle (especially with flip angles less that 45°), which makes careful selection of the partial flip angle critical to optimal MR imaging. The use of gradient-recalled echoes has a potential disadvantage as well, in that the information obtained is very sensitive to tissue magnetic-susceptibility effects and static-field inhomogeneity, and thus the information acquired is predominantly T_2^*-weighted. Tissue contrast can be controlled by adjusting the flip angle/gradient echo parameters. T_1-weighting decreases (and spin density weighting increases) as the flip angle is reduced. Relative short TR intervals provide a substantial degree of T_2^*-weighting and increasing the TE further increases T_2^* contrast. Typical settings and contrast weighting for TR/TE/flip angle are: 300/13/65 (T_1-weighting) 300/45/

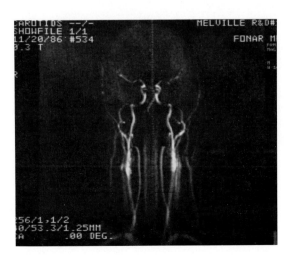

FIG. 6.37. A coronal head projection MRI sequence using a small-tip-angle/gradient-recalled-echo technique. The carotid arteries are seen well in this coronal projection image. (Courtesy of the FONAR Co. 0.3 T permanent magnet.)

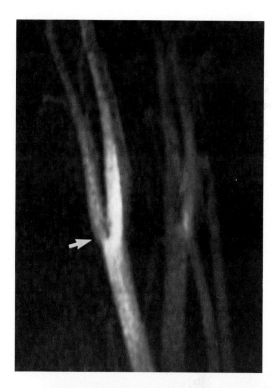

FIG. 6.38. Projection MRI angiogram of the left carotid artery (*arrow*) obtained with a selective blood-tagging inversion-recovery method. Blood flowing into the imaged region is tagged by a 180° inversion excitation for one of two images acquired. This results in a different signal on subtraction. The field of view is 9 × 12 cm and the image matrix 128 × 256; the acquisition time was approximately 4 min. The right carotid is less well seen because the surface coil used in this experiment was placed over the right carotid. (Courtesy of D. Nishimura and A. Macovski.)

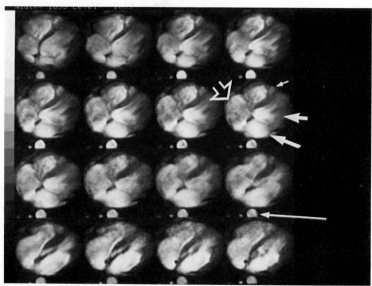

FIG. 6.39. Sixteen sequential cardiac images from a small-tip-angle/gradient-recalled-echo cine MRI angiogram. The images represent sequential cardiac cycles and the use of multiphasic acquisition developed by General Electric. The structures indicated are (from the longest to the shortest *solid arrows*): aorta, left atrium, left ventricle, and right ventricle, and the *open arrow* indicates the right atrium. The imaging sequence moves from left to right and indicates a diastole through systole and return to diastole. It is difficult to demonstrate the dynamic quality of these studies with static images; however, significant information is available in viewing a loop presentation of this material. (Courtesy of the General Electric Co.)

12 (T_2*-weighting); 400/13/10 (density-weighting). Chemical shift effects (artifacts) occur with these techniques due to the varying resonant frequencies of fat constituents and water. Depending on the TE, protons of different constituents may be in or out-of-phase resulting in diminished signal from fat or boundary zone signal loss between fat (CH_2 component) and water bearing tissues due to partial voluming of in and-out-of-phase protons (Fig. 6.40). Nevertheless, these small-flip-angle/field-echo techniques provide excellent static-tissue suppression and high-intensity signals from moving blood (Fig. 6.37).

Another interesting time-of-flight approach developed by Nishimura and Macovski utilizes a modified inversion-recovery sequence that allows subtraction angiography by varying the time-of-flight affects of flowing blood into a body region and projection imaging. A selective 180° excitation inverts different regions between measurements to isolate flow in both directions. The method thus yields a subtraction arteriogram that is based on controlled time-of-flight effects and blood tagging by manipulating the magnetic history of the tissue. The basic time-of-flight effects in imaging are signal loss due to washout of blood from an excited region and signal enhancement due to unsaturated blood flowing in. The selective inversion-recovery method switches the wash-in effect off and on to produce the different signals from blood. The directional effect is controlled by changing the region inverted by a selective 180° excitation. This method thus provides one-way directional sensitivity

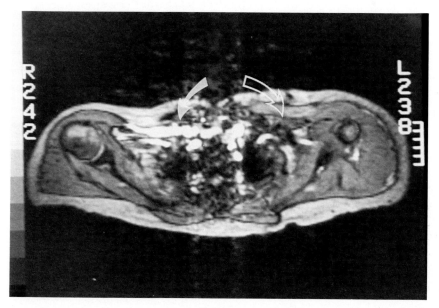

FIG. 6.40. A small-flip-angle (7°) gradient-recalled-echo axial sequence at the thoracic inlet in a patient suspected of having left subclavian and axillary vein occlusion. A venogram was attempted, but without success, and the MR image obtained reveals a patent right subclavian artery (*solid arrow*) and a completely occluded subclavian and axillary vein on the left (*open arrow*). Even though there is considerable artifact in this image, it is diagnostic of occlusion in the left subclavian and axillary vein.

to separate arterial flow from venous flow and, within limits, can image flow passing obliquely (or perpendicular) to the imaging plane. This is a distinct advantage over gradient-based methods of flow imaging, which can be blind to flow perpendicular to the gradient direction (Fig. 6.38). Both static and cine time-of-flight techniques can be used to evaluate other medical conditions such as vascular thrombosis and cardiac hemodynamic function (Figs. 6.39 and 6.40).

Flow-Dependent Phase-Shift Imaging

Motion- or flow-dependent phase-shift imaging is based on the fact that signal from moving protons can be made to undergo a phase shift that is directly proportional to the velocity of the protons. Phase-shift imaging differs from time-of-flight imaging in two important ways: (1) Imaging planes are selected that are longitudinal to the vessel of interest. Thus, flow is detected as it courses through the plane (or projection image). Vessel morphology is more accurately assessed in this approach than from cross-sectional imaging. (2) In phase-shift imaging, flow sensitivity is mediated by the phase of the NMR signal rather than by its amplitude or magnitude.

Gradient waveforms generally are used to encode velocity by means of phase-

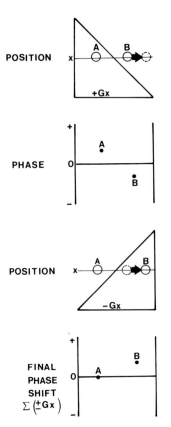

FIG. 6.41. The method of phase-angle encoding of flow and static-tissue suppression is initiated by applying a gradient ($+$Gx) and considering two structures—one static (A) and one moving (B) along the line indicated by position x. The sequence is initiated by applying a gradient ($+$Gx) that produces phase angles for both A and B, as indicated at phase one. Subsequently, a gradient is applied in the reverse direction ($-$Gx). A, which has not moved, has complete phase cancellation as a result of the positive and negative gradients having been applied. However, B, which moved from its initial position to a position farther to the right along the x axis, has not had complete phase cancellation and, in this case, has a remaining final phase shift, as indicated in the final phase-shift diagram. The imaginary image (i.e., an image in which the gray scale represents the phase angle of the tissue within the voxel) can be displayed as a gray-scale representation, with those tissues having zero phase being completely cancelled. Structures having a nonzero phase as the result of motion are assigned a gray-scale value representing their phase angles. One problem with this technique is that 360° multiples of the same phase angle will be assigned to the same step in the gray scale, and additional processing is necessary to resolve this type of problem.

shift information. The simplest type of gradient waveform that will produce this effect is shown in Fig. 6.41. Point A represents a stationary object, and B is an object flowing parallel, with the bipolar gradients labeled $+Gx$ and $-Gx$. The bipolar gradients consist of a negative lobe followed by a positive lobe, and they are equal in amplitude and duration. The stationary object (A) will experience a phase shift during the first lobe of this waveform that will depend on its position along x. It will then experience an exactly equal and opposite phase shift during the second lobe of the waveform, so that its net phase shift will be zero.

An object that is moving along the x axis (B) will also experience a phase shift during the first lobe of the waveform, followed by an opposite phase shift during the second lobe. B, however, has changed its position because of its velocity along the x axis and thus will experience a different phase shift at the time of the second lobe. The two phase shifts will not exactly cancel each other, and the moving proton will be left with a net phase shift that will be directly proportional to its velocity along x while the gradient waveform is applied. The amount of phase shift per centimeter per second is a function of the moment of a gradient waveform. One major advantage of this approach to flow imaging is that the instantaneous velocity of the protons can be calculated because the gradient waveform can be quite short in duration. There is thus a possibility of eliminating signal from stationary tissues that experience zero phase shift or very little phase shift. One major disadvantage of this approach is that it is strictly directional and is insensitive to flow perpendicular to the axis. As with time-of-flight techniques, turbulent flow can become quite confusing, and low signal or high signal may occur in areas of marked turbulence. Other sources of phase shift are also a problem, especially the eddy currents induced in the magnet by the gradients themselves. Such phase shifts are indistinguishable from phase shifts caused by motion. Another potential problem is that the pixel intensity in the final image is a sinusoidal function of velocity. Thus, although relative phase can be assigned with some certainty, whether a given intensity is proportional to a flow at 2π, or 4π, or any other 360° phase multiple cannot be ascertained from the data.

An interesting approach to using flow-dependent phase shifts has been the phase-display approach of Wideen. In order to make proton phase shifts readily visible, a special phase-sensitive image reconstruction is used. A phase-display image is produced in which tissues of constant phase are represented by black and white "zebra stripes." The position of each stripe indicates the velocity of the protons at that location. Straight stripes indicate stationary protons, whereas displacement of the stripes indicates flow. In order to obtain these images, a set of diastolic and systolic phase images is acquired and then subtracted.

MRI data are stored as complex numbers in the computer memory, and the phase-display images are obtained by additional processing of the complex-number set. Complex numbers are the two numbers in a Cartesian coordinate system that define a point in a plane. Thus, it takes two ordinary (real) numbers to specify one complex number. The same point can be identified in polar-coordinates by use of a vector and an angle (phase angle) of elevation above some reference line (e.g., the abscissa), and these two sets of numbers can also be used to describe a complex number. Specifying the location of a complex number in a Cartesian or polar coordinate system involves specifying what are referred to as the real and imaginary parts. When the complex number is described in polar coordinates, it is specified by a magnitude M (real) and a phase (imaginary) angle (e.g., 30°). In MRI, the software initially constructs a complex number for each voxel and then calculates an ordinary one-dimensional number in order to assign a gray-scale rating to the voxel. The magnitude M of the polar representation determines the image intensity in conventional MRI. No phase information is represented in this type of image display. Phase-display imaging employs software to process the complex numbers and create images in which the image intensity (gray scale) is directly proportional to the imaginary part of the complex number or, in other words, the phase angle of the magnetic vector.

The many approaches to flow imaging are in a continual state of flux. New refinements and entirely new approaches are still being developed. The MR signal is also sensitive to diffusion and brownian motion within fluids, and some attempts have been made to derive diagnostic information from the diffusion and brownian-motion characteristics of body tissues. At this point, the clinical utility of flow imaging is uncertain, and perhaps the best strategy is to remain skeptical until clear clinical applications have been established. The sensitivity and specificity of these approaches have not been well established. Imaging coronary vessels and delineating the importance of collaterals, both in the heart and around occlusions in peripheral vessels, are not currently part of the imaging capabilities of MR angiography. Dealing with turbulence and distinguishing between signals due to turbulence, plaque, and vessel occlusion are likely to be difficult problems to solve with the currently available techniques. In addition, conventional X-ray angiography is a relatively safe method that is well understood and provides very high spatial resolution and a minimum number of artifacts. Carotids, jugulars, and other peripheral vessels are also evaluated on a regular basis using Doppler ultrasound. It probably will be some time before the exact relationships between MRI and other types of vascular diagnostic options are clearly established.

Clotted Blood

Considerable research effort has been expended to find MRI markers for differentiating between edema and hemorrhage and also determining the ages of hemorrhages and hematomas. Because of the magnetic-susceptibility differences at low and high field strengths, this type of differential analysis appears to be possible only at high field strengths (>1 T). Conceptually, there are several stages of hemorrhage, including a progression of hemoglobin from an early preponderance of oxyhemoglobin through deoxygenation to deoxyhemoglobin and surrounding edema and, subsequently, methemoglobin within intact cells and eventually within lysed red blood cells. On conversion to hemosiderin, the macrophages then phagocytose the hemosiderin granules, and it is this that represents the long-standing end stage of hematoma formation.

During the early stages of hemorrhage there is little T_1 or T_2 effect (Table 6.1). With the formation of methemoglobin, either within or outside of red blood cells,

TABLE 6.1. *Hemorrhage evolution and resulting T_1 and T_2 changes*

Stage	T_1	T_2
Oxyhemoglobin	0	0
Deoxyhemoglobin	0	↓
Methemoglobin (in RBC)	↓	↓
Methemoglobin (free)	↓	↑
Hemosiderin	0	↓ ↓
Edema	↑	↑

there is a modest shortening of T_1. T_2 changes are more complex in that there is shortening of T_2 relaxation times associated with deoxyhemoglobin and with methemoglobin contained within red blood cells. However, on red blood cell lysis there is a significant prolongation of T_2. At this stage in hematoma evolution, typically 1 week to 1 month of age, one sees a shortened T_1 and a prolonged T_2, generally recognized as intense signal on both T_1- and T_2-weighted images. With the formation of hemosiderin, however, there is considerable shortening of T_2 relaxation again. Conversely, surrounding edema generally prolongs both T_1 and T_2 and on this basis can be differentiated from the hemorrhage itself (Figs. 6.42–6.44) (see Chapter 5 regarding gray scale in MRI).

Of course, exact assignment of these various stages to the gray-scale image will depend critically on the imaging sequence used (i.e., TR, TI, TE, B_0). In addition, the small-flip-angle/gradient-recalled-echo techniques, which have a significant T_2^* or magnetic-susceptibility component, will produce images that are very sensitive to the superparamagnetic-iron content in the tissue.

MRI OF THE ABDOMEN AND PELVIS

Following the example developed in CT scanning, MRI evaluation of the abdomen and pelvis has proceeded somewhat more slowly than have the applications developed for neurological diseases. In part, this is because the available scanner time has been taken up by the clearly superior applications of MRI in neurological diseases. Perhaps a more important consideration is that for the abdomen and pelvis there are several other technologies available that have been shown to be good diagnostic procedures and, in many cases, relatively less expensive than MRI procedures. However, the availability of ultrasound, CT, intravenous pyelography, barium studies, and plain radiography does not provide the entire explanation. One of the more difficult technical problems has been the control of motion artifacts. The technical problem is considerably more difficult than that of controlling phase and motion artifacts in the vertebral column, because the direction and expected velocity of motion are substantially more variable than those encountered in oscillatory CSF pulsations. Nevertheless, there has been considerable progress, and MRI is taking its place as an important diagnostic technique for evaluation of the abdomen.

Cardiovascular and respiratory artifacts have been particularly troublesome in the

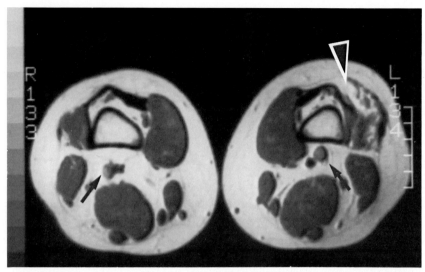

A

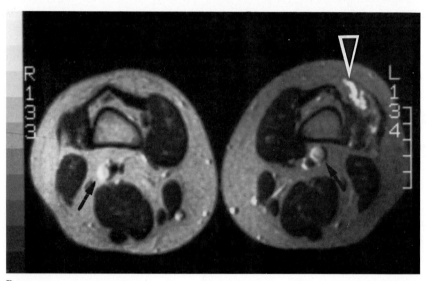

B

FIG. 6.42. Axial MR images obtained for evaluation of a patient with a painful swelling above the left patella. A CT scan had revealed an abnormal mass in this area, but on MRI examination a large hematoma was found in the vastus lateralis muscle (*black-and-white arrowhead*). High-intensity signal on the first and second echoes suggests the presence of methemoglobin in lysed red blood cells. This would indicate the lesion to be 1 week to a few weeks in age. These images also illustrate flow-related contrast enhancement of flowing blood and even-echo rephasing, with high-intensity signal coming from the femoral veins on the second echo of this sequence (*black arrows*) (1.5 T, 1500/25/50, 256 × 256, NEX 2, FOV 32, Skip 20%).

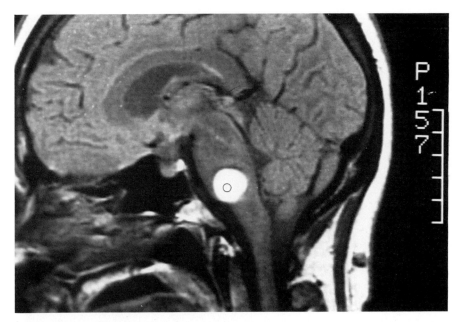

A

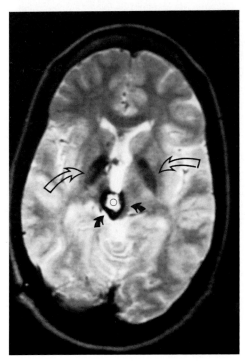

B

FIG. 6.43. Sagittal (**A**, 1500/20) T_1-weighted image and axial (**B**, 2000/75) T_2-weighted image from a patient known to have a brainstem hematoma. The presence centrally within this lesion of high-intensity signal on the images (**A, B,** *circle*) indicates the presence of free methemoglobin. Surrounding hemosiderin is not well seen on the sagittal more T_1-weighted image because of its limited effect on T_1 relaxation; however, in the more T_2-weighted axial image, the hemosiderin is well defined (*black curved arrows*). Incidentally noted is another iron collection in the globus pallidus (*open curved arrows*). Iron deposits can be normally associated with aging or can be abnormally associated with degenerative disorders such as Parkinson's disease.

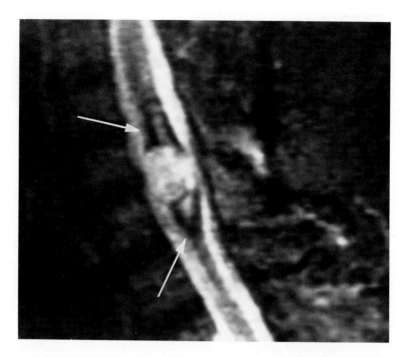

FIG. 6.44. Sagittal MR image, heavily T$_2$-weighted (1.5 T, 2000/80), from a patient with a neoplasm and associated old hemorrhage of the thoracic spinal cord. The low-intensity signal above and below the body of the mass indicates hemosiderin deposits (*arrows*). Mottling within the tumor is due to magnetic susceptibility effects.

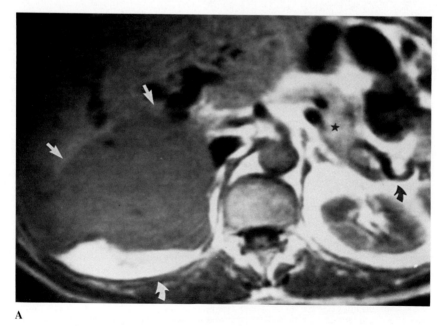

A

FIG. 6.45. Axial T$_1$-weighted (**A**, 800/20) and T$_2$-weighted (**B**, 1500/75) MR images from a patient with a hemangioma of the liver, and two-on-one pre-contrast CT scan (**C**) and post-contrast CT scan (**D**) of the same area. The hemangioma (*white arrows*) is shown to have a relatively long T$_1$ (**A**) and relatively long T$_2$ (**B**).

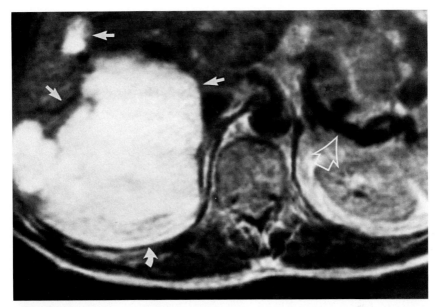

B

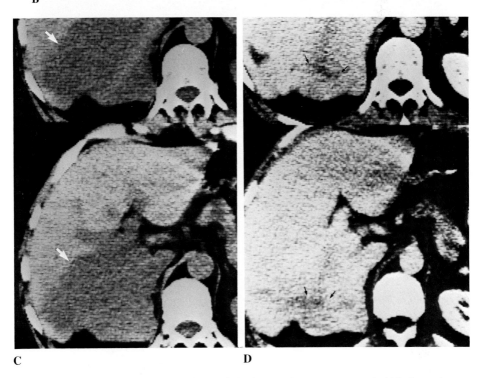

C   D

FIG. 6.45. (*continued*) A second focus of the hemangioma appears anteriorly (*arrow*) on the T$_2$-weighted image. The hemangioma characteristically partially fills in (*small black arrows*) after intravenous administration of contrast material on CT examination (**C & D**). A second component of the hemangioma is seen posteriorly (*curved arrow*). This area shows complex behavior on MRI evaluation, and the high intensities on both T$_1$- and T$_2$-weighted images suggest areas of hemorrhage. Also note the pancreas (*star*) and splenic artery (*curved black arrow*) and vein (*open white arrow*).

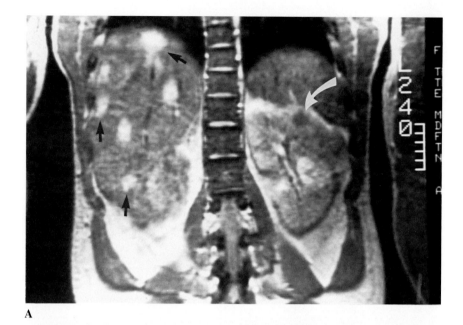

A

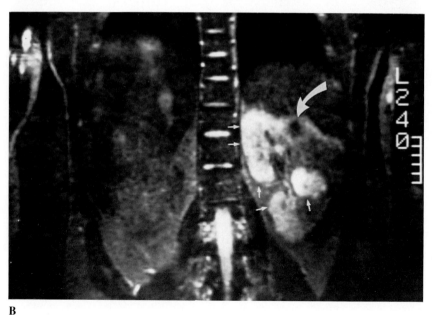

B

FIG. 6.46. Coronal MR images from a 30-year-old man with tuberous sclerosis (**A**, 1,500/ 40; **B**, 1,500/80). Angiomyolipomas in the liver are predominantly composed of fat (*black arrows*—three are marked) and show a characteristic decrease in signal on the second echo. The lesions within the kidney are more heterogeneous—some are composed primarily of muscle (*curved white arrow*), whereas others are predominantly cystic (*white arrows*). The high-intensity nucleus pulposus on the second echo is characteristic of a younger person, and there is even-echo enhancement in the vessels inferiorly in the right side of the pelvis.

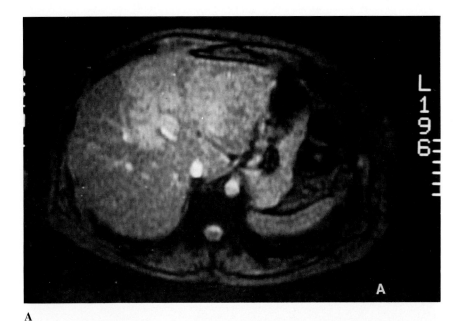

A

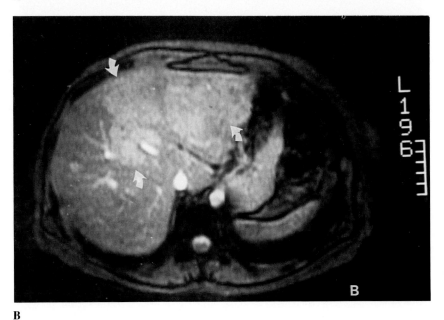

B

FIG. 6.47. Axial images using a small-tip-angle/gradient-recalled-echo technique in a patient with breast cancer metastatic to the liver. This series illustrates fast scanning and the
effects of varying tip angle and short TR values in liver evaluation. Images **A, B** (hepatic
breast metastases, *curved arrows*), and **C** were obtained using a sequence of TR = 40
msec, TE = 12 msec, and 5°, 9°, and 15° tip angles, respectively. Image **D,** for comparison,
employed TR = 22 msec, TE = 12 msec, and a tip angle of 9°. Image **E** is from a fast
inversion-recovery technique.

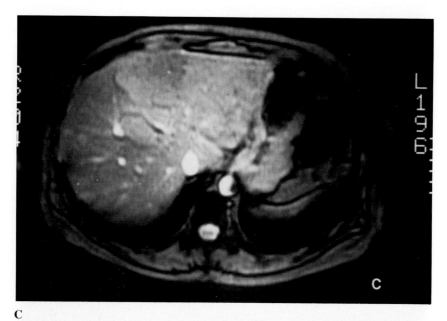

C

D

FIG. 6.47. (*continued*). Note that although the signal-to-noise ratio increases from **A** through **C** (because of the increasing transverse magnetization as the tissue magnetic vector is progressively tipped from 5° to 15°), detectability of the metastases within the liver decreases in **C** because of an increased signal emanating from normal liver as compared with that from the metastases. Image **D**, using a shorter TR interval, thus allowing less longitudinal relaxation, should be compared with image **B** and is noteworthy because in spite of its higher noise level, related to the shorter TR interval, conspicuity or contrast resolution of the metastases in the liver is greater in image **D** than in image **B** possibly because of the longer T_1 values in the liver, however. Magnetic susceptibility and flow also are reflected in these images and undoubtedly contribute to the higher (whiter) cancer signal.

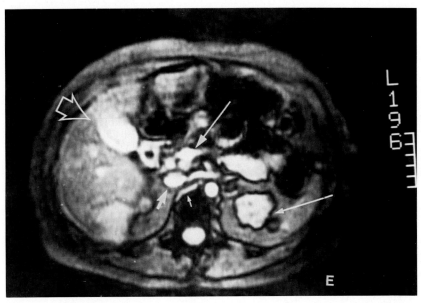

E

FIG. 6.47. (*continued*). Motion produces a white appearance using this small-tip-angle/ gradient-recalled-echo technique, and blood vessels are well seen, as are the metastases within the liver. The entire liver was imaged using TR = 40 msec, TE = 12 msec, and 9° angle. Image **E,** using a short-TI inversion-recovery technique, was obtained at the level of the left renal vein for comparison. Indicated are the gallbladder (*open arrow*) and, in order of increasing arrow length, the right renal artery, the inferior vena cava (with left renal vein crossing over the aorta and superior mesenteric artery crossing just anterior to this), the confluence of the portal vein and splenic vein, and the left kidney, with a cyst on the posterior lateral aspect of the upper pole of the left kidney. The high intensity anterior to the left kidney is due to fluid moving within the stomach. The dome of the right kidney is also seen. Note the edge enhancement of the bounce-point artifact often seen with this imaging sequence.

upper abdomen when scanning the lower lung fields, liver, spleen, and pancreas. In some cases, special gating procedures and respiratory-motion compensation techniques are not necessary to obtain an adequate examination (Fig. 6.45). However, in general, MRI studies in this area are best undertaken with at least some form of respiratory compensation (Fig. 6.46). Short TI inversion recovery sequences and fast scanning has been useful in evaluating the liver (Fig. 6.47). Small-tip-angle/ gradient-recalled-echo techniques have specifically been useful in evaluating vascular patency in the abdomen. For example, these techniques have been useful in establishing the presence or absence of renal vein thrombosis or tumor invasion in the presence of renal carcinoma (Fig. 6.48). Improved spatial resolution has also enabled evaluation of the adrenals (Fig. 6.49), and the improved sensitivity of both T_1- and T_2-weighted images has been shown repeatedly to provide information not available on conventional CT scanning (Fig. 6.50).

MRI evaluation of the lower abdomen and pelvis has proceeded more rapidly, and imaging quality has been superior in these areas because there is relatively less motion in the lower abdomen and pelvis. The sensitivity of T_1-, T_2,- and flow-

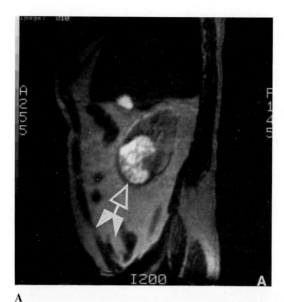

FIG. 6.48. A series of MR images from a patient known to have renal cell carcinoma of the right kidney being evaluated for a question of right renal vein thrombosis. A sagittal MR image was obtained (**A**, TR = 1,500 msec, TE = 70 msec) that revealed renal cell carcinoma involving the lower pole of the right kidney (*open arrow*). A small-tip-angle/gradient/recalled-echo sequence was obtained first axially at the level of the left renal vein (**B**), illustrating flowing blood as a high-intensity signal. Indicated are the left renal vein (*curved black arrow*) and artery (*straight black arrow*), inferior vena cava (*star*), aorta (*bullet*), and left renal vein (*curved white arrow*).

A

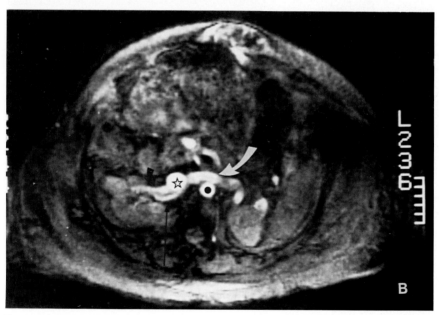

B

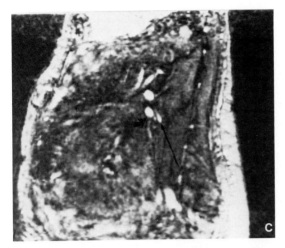

C

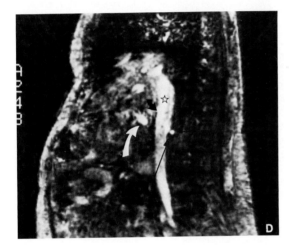

D

FIG. 6.48. (*continued*). The origin of the superior mesenteric vein is seen just anterior to the junction of the left renal vein and inferior vena cava. A sagittal sequence beginning from the hilum of the right kidney to just to the left of the aorta was then obtained using the same technique (**C–G**). The right renal vein and artery are seen in **C** (*curved and straight black arrows,* respectively). Image **D** is sagittal, obtained at the level of the inferior vena cava (*star*), with anatomy as follows: the right renal vein entering the cava (*curved black arrow*), the left renal vein entering the cava above the right renal artery passing posterior to the inferior vena cava (*straight black arrow*). The splenic vein and superior mesenteric vein confluence is seen on this image (*curved white arrow*) and on image E anterior to the IVC. The renal veins and arteries are shown to be patient by this series of images.

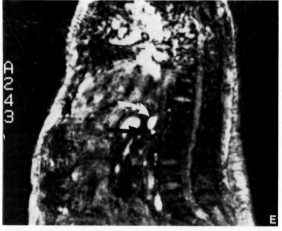

E

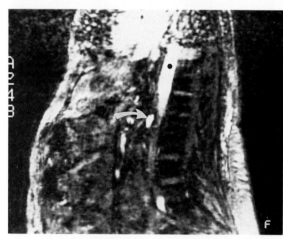

F

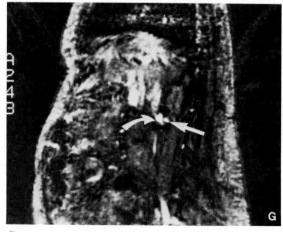

G

FIG. 6.48. (*continued*). A sagittal image (**E**) obtained between the inferior vena cava and aorta reveals the right renal artery (*straight black arrow*) and the left renal vein (*curved white arrow*). The sagittal image obtained at the level of the abdominal aorta (*bullet*) reveals the left renal vein (*curved arrow*), passing anterior to the aorta; the right renal artery has entered the aorta, and the left has not taken its origin at this level. The sagittal image obtained just lateral to the aorta (**G**) reveals the left renal vein (*curved arrow*) and artery (*straight arrow*). This sequence establishes the patency of both the right and left renal arteries and gives a clearer view of this patency than was obtained from the axial images. All images made with TR = 20 msec and TE = 12 msec.

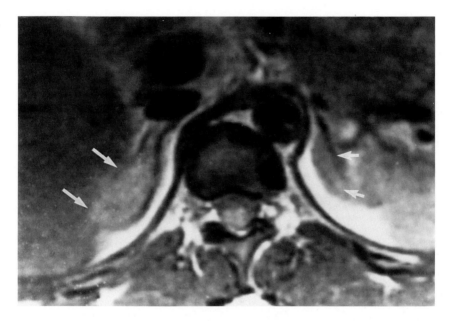

FIG. 6.49. Axial MR image obtained from a patient with Parkinson's disease (TR = 800 msec, TE = 24 msec) revealing bilateral adrenal hyperplasia (*arrows*).

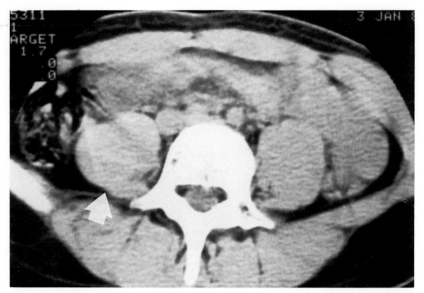

A

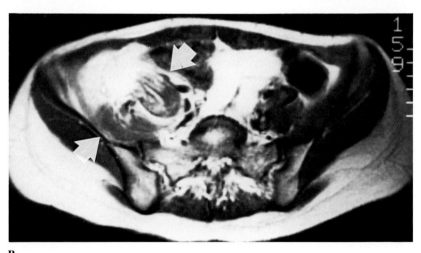

B

FIG. 6.50. A series of studies including an axial CT scan (**A**) and an MRI study consisting of a partial-saturation axial (**B,** TR = 800 msec, TE = 24 msec) and two sagittal (**C&D,** TR = 2,000 msec, TE = 40 and 80 msec) MR images from a 14-year-old female with recent onset of right-leg pain. The CT scan revealed some minimal psoas asymmetry (*white arrow*). On the MRI study 2 weeks later, this area was found to have been involved with a nonosseous Ewing's sarcoma that was considerably larger than estimated by the CT scan (*white arrows*). The inverted U-shaped high-intensity signal to the left of the tumor is a loop of bowel. The neoplast can be seen to have a relatively long T_2 on the sagittal images. The psoas muscle posterior to the tumor at this level is not invaded. However, a large extension of the tumor does project anterior to the psoas across the inguinal ligament.

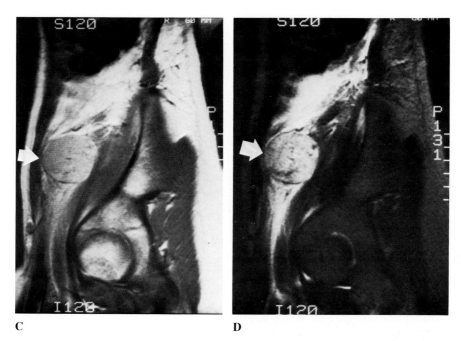

C   D

FIG. 6.50. continued.

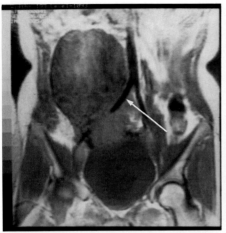

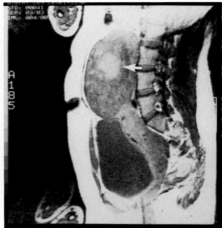

A   B

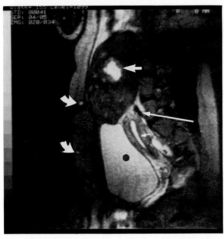

C

FIG. 6.51. Coronal partial-saturation (**A**), sagittal partial-saturation (**B**), and T$_2$-weighted spin-echo (**C**) MR images from a patient who presented complaining of an abdominal mass. The MRI study reveals a huge lyomyoma involving the entire mid-abdomen arising from the superior right aspect of the uterus and crossing anterior to the right iliac artery (*long white arrow*). The study reveals that the fibroid has a hemorrhagic center, with a signal of relatively high intensity on both the T$_1$ and T$_2$-weighted images (*middle-size arrow*). The endometrium and zona basalis show similar characteristic signal in **C** (*small arrow*). Abdominal veins in the anterior abdominal wall have undergone even-echo enhancement (*curved white arrows*). The bladder shows the characteristics of a liquid with rapidly tumbling small molecules, although there is some motion, and spin dispersion is noted near the base of the bladder on the T$_2$-weighted image (*bullet*). (1.5 T; **A&B**, 600/20; **C**, 2000/80.)

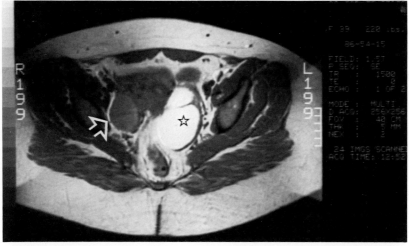

A

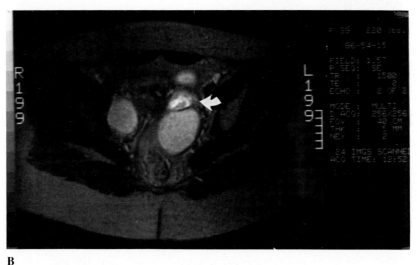

B

FIG. 6.52. First- and second-echo axial (**A&B**, 1500/25/75; 1 ⁻) and coronal (**C&D**, 2000/25/75) MR images from a 39-year-old woman with premenstrual pain and abnormal findings on pelvic examination. This study illustrates the differential information that can be obtained from an MRI study. A CT scan obtained from this patient prior to MRI revealed only abnormal pelvic masses, but was unable to further elucidate the cause or further characterize the lesions. This MRI study, however, reveals the presence of uterine fibroids (*long white arrows*), a right adnexal cyst that was found to be nonepithelialized at surgery (*open arrow*), and a complex mass in the left adnexal (*star*), with areas showing high-intensity signal on both first and second echoes characteristic of blood (*curved white arrow*). This was found to be an area of hemorrhagic endometriosis at the time of surgery. Evaluating MR images can be facilitated even without completely understanding the pulsing sequences and all of the input functions related to the gray scale by comparing known tissues to unknown structures.

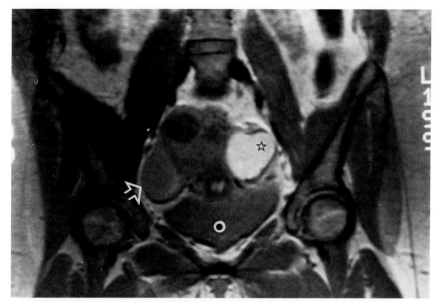

C

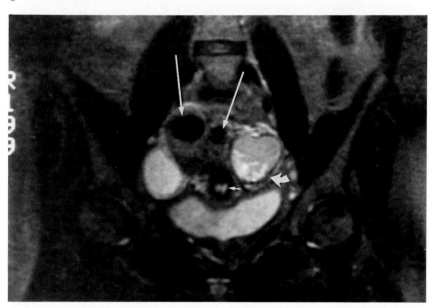

D

FIG. 6.52. (*continued*). In this case, the right adnexal abnormality has characteristics comparable to those seen within the bladder (*bullet*) and therefore must represent a cyst, whereas the left adnexal mass has components that perform like the menstrual blood within the endometrial cavity (*short white arrow*). Similarly, the low-intensity spherical lesions within the uterus yield signal intensities on both first and second echoes comparable to those for the psoas and iliacus muscle (*long white arrows*) and were found to be fibroids. Also note, on the second echo, even-echo enhancement in the hemorrhoidal vessels, and a left external iliac vein. There is a small amount of fluid in the hip joints bilaterally, seen as a high-intensity echo on the second-echo coronal view.

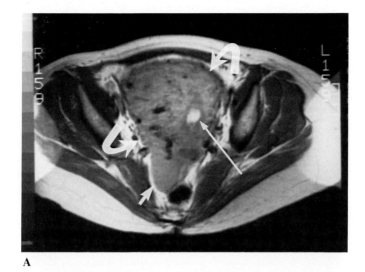

A

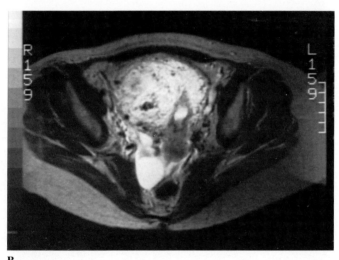

B

FIG. 6.53. Axial first- and second-echo MRI study at the level of the pelvis (**A&B**, 1.5 T, 1500/25/75) in a patient known to have choriocarcinoma. The choriocarcinoma nearly completely fills the pelvis (*curved arrows*). There is a right adnexal cyst (*short arrow*), and zona basalis in the endometrial cavity is seen in an anteverted uterus (*long white arrow*). The signal intensity within the tumor reveals very little hemorrhage in this mass, as compared with the case in Fig. 6.52. This can be discerned by comparing the signal intensity with that for the right adnexal cyst. The low-intensity features within the tumor are related to flow voids within feeding arteries and draining veins. Even-echo slow-flow vascular enhancement is seen in the adnexa and in the fat of the anterior lower abdominal wall. (Courtesy of C. L. Carrol.)

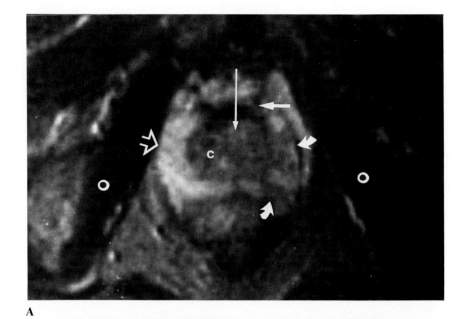

A

B   C

FIG. 6.54. Magnified axial MRI (**A,** TR = 2,000 msec, TE = 80 msec) in a patient with prostatic carcinoma, sagittal view from another patient (**B,** TR = 800 msec, TE = 25 msec) with prostatic carcinoma who had been treated with radiation therapy, and a magnified sagittal view from a third patient (**C,** TR = 800 msec, TE = 20 msec) with metastases to the lower vertebral column. The normal and abnormal anatomic features of the prostate are well illustrated in image **A**: the high-intensity peripheral zone (*open arrow*), the somewhat lower intensity of the central zone (**C**) and the somewhat higher intensity of the periurethral zone (*long arrow*), and the fibromuscular band (*intermediate-size arrow*). The prostatic cancer has broken through the peripheral zone on the left (*curved arrows*), but has not invaded the obturator internus muscles (*bullets*). In **B,** the patient has been treated with radiation therapy.

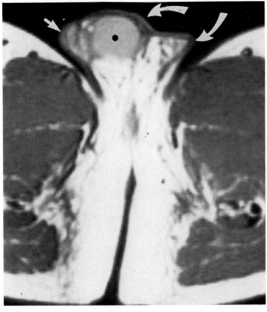

A

FIG. 6.55. Axial MRI studies of normal testicle (*bullet*) and epididymis (*straight arrow*). The left and right scrotal wall is also seen (*curved white arrows*) (**A**, 2,000/ 25; **B**, 2,000/70).

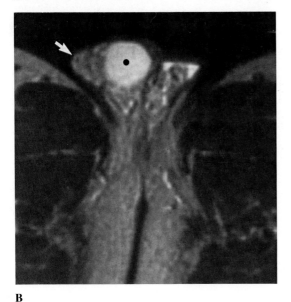

B

FIG. 6.54. (*continued*). The tumor is seen at the base of the bladder (*curved arrow*). The fatty replacement of the lower sacral bone marrow (*open black arrows*) is seen in contrast to the lower-intensity marrow in this patient, with some degenerative changes in the vertebral column (*straight black arrows*). The high-intensity fatty marrow can serve as a good indicator of subsequent metastatic disease to the vertebral column, as indicated in **C** (*curved black arrows*). The prostatic neoplasm is seen in the bladder base (*curved white arrow*), and there is significant bladder thickening in this patient (*short white arrows*).

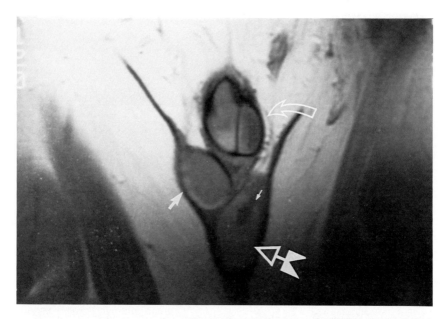

FIG. 6.56. Coronal MRI study of a patient with a prosthetic plastic right testicle (*large white arrow*). The left testicle is normal (*open arrow*), and the mediastinum testis (*small white arrow*) is seen superiorly in the normal left testicle. The paired corpora cavernosa are seen superiorly (*open curved arrow*).

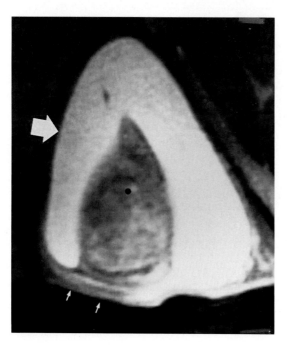

FIG. 6.57. A T₂-weighted (2,000/70) image from a patient with an embryonal cell carcinoma of the testicle (*bullet*). A large surrounding hydrocele is also seen (*large white arrow*). The various layers of the scrotal wall, including the dartos muscle, are identified inferiorly (*small white arrows*). (Courtesy of D. Sidenwurm.)

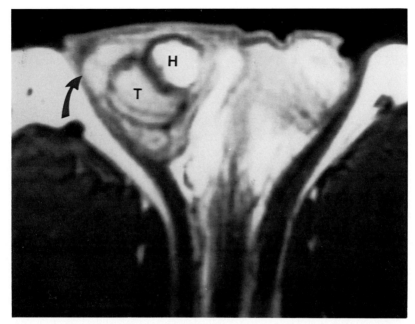

A

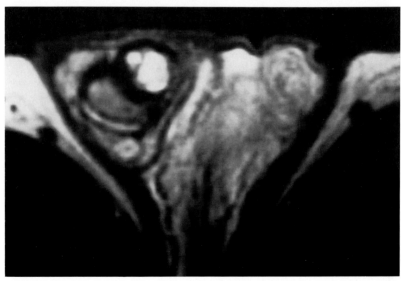

B

FIG. 6.58. Balanced (2,000/25) and T$_2$-weighted (2,000/70) axial MR images from a patient with a traumatic injury to the testicle. The testicle is atrophic (T), and a focus of hemorrhage is seen anteriorly (H). The surrounding low-intensity signal was related to hemosiderin. The epididymis is seen on both views (*curved black arrow*). The scrotal sack of the other testicle is seen, and there are flow-related artifacts in the spermatic cord just inferior to the atrophic testicle. (Courtesy of D. Sidenwurm.)

weighted images has provided excellent diagnostic information in evaluating both
normal anatomy and pathological conditions of the pelvis (Figs. 6.51–6.54). The
use of surface coils has also enabled evaluation of benign and malignant conditions
of the testicles (Figs. 6.55–6.58).

MRI OF THE JOINTS AND EXTREMITIES

MRI of the joints and extremities is revolutionizing the practice of musculoskeletal imaging. Many of the early concerns about little or no signal emanating from
cortical bone have given way to excitement regarding the opportunities for imaging
cartilage and the bone marrow. Abnormalities that increase the water content of

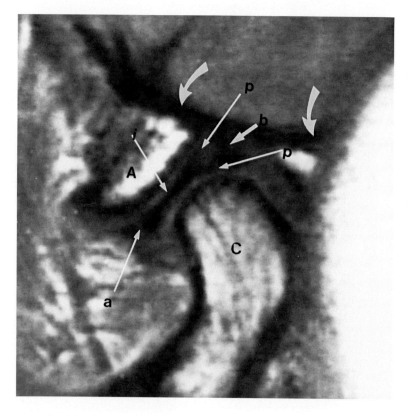

FIG. 6.59. Normal MRI examination of the left temporomandibular joint in an asymptomatic
volunteer (1,500/25). This is a closed-mouth view through the middle of the condyle of the
mandible. Indicated are the marrow within the mandibular condyle (C) and marrow within the
articular tubercle of the temporal bone (A), the subdivisions of the meniscus, including the
anterior band (a), the intermediate zone (i), and the superior and inferior divisions of the
posterior band (p) where they join the bilaminar zone (b). The curvilinear low-intensity signal
above the bilaminar zone (*curved white arrows*) is the thin bony plate of the temporal bone
in the middle cranial fossa (the arrows overlap the temporal lobe in this area).

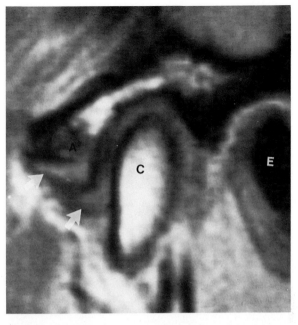

A

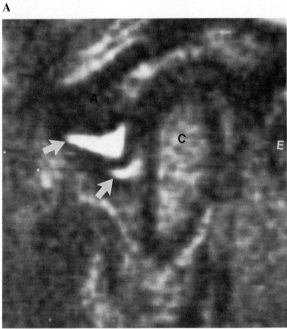

B

FIG. 6.60. Sagittal MRI study (**A,** 1,500/25; **B,** 1,500/70) in a patient with pain on opening the jaw, performed in the closed-mouth position. Effusion in the temporomandibular joint is seen in both views (*arrows*) and shows the characteristic increased signal intensity on the T$_2$-weighted image. The anteriorly displaced meniscus is outlined by the effusions. The articular eminence (A) and the marrow within the mandibular condyle (C), as well as the external auditory canal (E), are indicated. The patient's displacement was reduced with a minimum of 10 mm of open-mouth positioning and would have been missed had only an image with slightly open mouth been obtained. (Courtesy of J. Drace.)

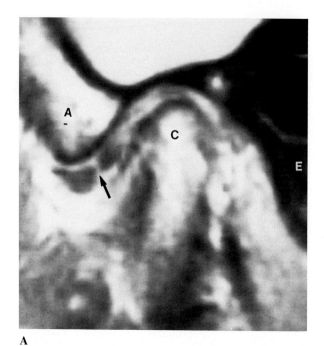

A

B

FIG. 6.61. Sagittal MR images from a patient with severe pain in the left temporomandibular joint (**A,** 1,500/25; **B,** 1,500/70). The MRI study reveals multiple perforations of the meniscus (*arrows*). The patient had limited range of motion, and increased signal intensity in the bilaminar zone (over the condyle, C) indicated edema and inflammation. Marrow in the articular eminence (A) is indicated. The low-density structure surrounding the articular eminence is the cortical bone.

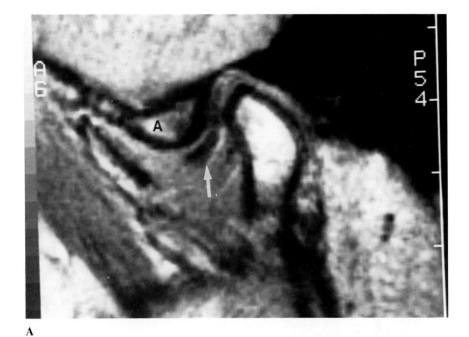

A

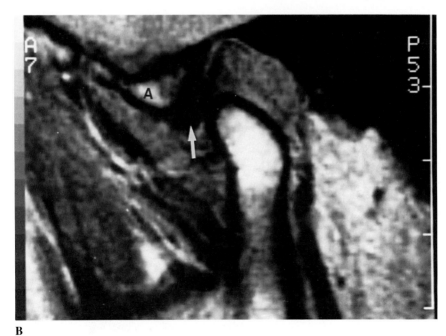

B

FIG. 6.62. Closed-mouth (**A**) and open-mouth (**B**) sagittal MR images from a patient with pain in the left temporomandibular joint. On these partial-saturation views (800/20), note increased signal intensity from the intermediate and posterior zones of the meniscus, indicating degenerative change. On the open-mouth view, the left side opens very little (note that the condyle does not pass beyond the articular eminence), and the meniscus does not reduce. This lack of change of position of the meniscus and the severe degeneration near the bilaminar zone indicate possible disruption of the meniscus.

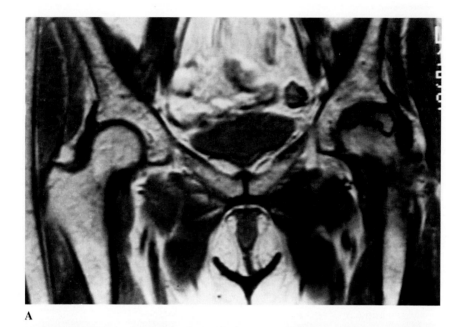

A

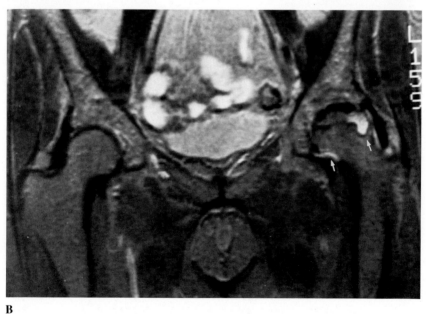

B

FIG. 6.63. Coronal MRI studies from a 23-year-old woman with aseptic necrosis of the left femoral head (**A,** 1,000/40; **B,** 1,000/80). Note the anatomic asymmetry and decreased signal emanating from the marrow in the left femoral head. Also note on the T$_2$-weighted image (**B**) an effusion in the left hip joint (*arrows*). Comparison of the signal intensities in these two images with that for the bladder would indicate that the high-intensity signal in the femoral head represents fluid or a cyst. Also note even-echo enhancement in the vessels superior to the pubic symphysis.

cortical bone, such as fractures or metastases to the cortex, are conspicuous because of the surrounding low-intensity signal from normal cortical bone. Surface coils have greatly improved the spatial resolution in the temporomandibular joint (Figs. 6.59–6.62). Various conditions involving the hip, especially aseptic necrosis, have shown early diagnostic indications, such as the double-ring phenomenon (black and white intensities on MR images), that indicate very early aseptic necrosis (Fig. 6.63). The knee has been extensively studied, and MRI promises to be the noninvasive technique of choice for preoperative evaluation of various conditions of the knee joint (Figs. 6.64–6.67). Involvement of the bone marrow, as has been described in previous chapters, is also clearly evident on MRI (Fig. 6.68), even when findings on plain radiographs and CT scans are normal.

ARTIFACTS IN CLINICAL MRI

Artifacts can arise from a great variety of sources pertaining both to characteristics of the scanner and to characteristics of the patient and the interaction between the two. Artifacts can degrade images sufficiently to cause inaccurate diagnoses. An understanding of artifacts is important if the physician is to avoid errors in clinical diagnosis. The most common artifacts are due to magnetic inhomogeneity in the B_0 or B_1 field, and surface coils intrinsically have local-field falloff. Many of the artifacts discussed are illustrated in images in other chapters, and they are indicated where appropriate.

Motion Artifacts

Patient-motion artifacts due to breathing and cardiovascular and CSF pulsations probably are the most frequently encountered artifacts in MRI, and they are capable of causing image degradation and diagnostic difficulties. The phase axis is very sensitive to motion. Ghost images appear as a complex series of both positive and negative image replicas in the phase-encoded direction (Fig. 6.69). Relatively slow laminar flow often manifests increased signal intensity in vessels on even-numbered echoes. A signal is most intense if the even echo is an integral multiple of the first echo, producing a full 360° rotation, and symmetrical TE times are used. This phenomenon is due to incomplete rephasing of the transverse magnetization vectors following an odd-number 180° pulse. Nearly complete rephasing occurs subsequently on even-numbered 180° pulses. This phenomenon is still flow-sensitive, and on multiple-echo sequences, if the protons are washed out of the excited slice, signal falloff may be seen even on subsequent even echoes (Fig. 6.70). Motion in the cervical thoracic CSF can be very confusing on MR images. The pulsatile CSF flow creates a modulation with the phase-encoding gradients. In addition, areas of pulsatile flow also undergo phase dispersion and turbulent flow in the CSF as it courses around the dentate ligament, or around other obstructions in the spinal canal (Fig. 6.71).

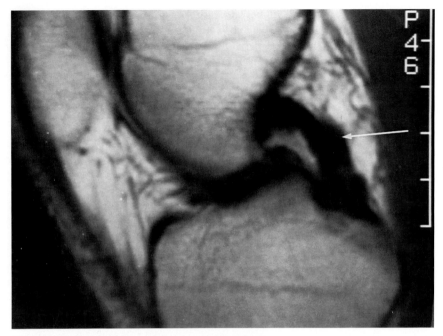

A

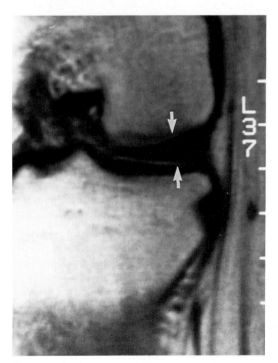

FIG. 6.64. Sagittal (**A**) and coronal (**B**) views (1,500/20) of normal knee joints, for comparison with the following pathological studies. The sagittal view is obtained at the level of the posterior cruciate ligament (*arrow*), and the coronal view is a detail of the medial meniscus (*short arrows*).

B

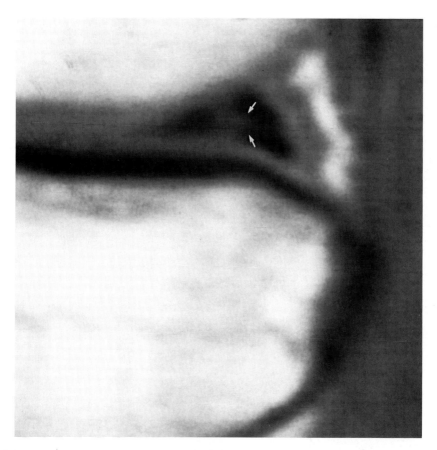

FIG. 6.65. Coronal-detail MRI of a stellate tear in the medial meniscus (*arrows*).

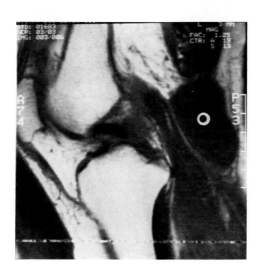

FIG. 6.66. Sagittal MRI study from a patient with painless swelling posterior to the knee joint (1,500/40). The study reveals a Baker's cyst (*bullet*).

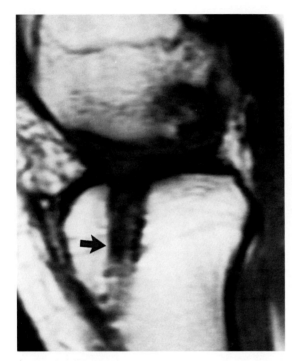

A

FIG. 6.67. Sagittal (**A**) and coronal (**B**) MRI studies (1,500/20) from a patient with a previously ruptured anterior cruciate ligament and reimplantation of the quadriceps tendon through the tibial plateau (*black arrows*). There is considerable joint effusion (*white arrows*), and neither collateral ligament is normal.

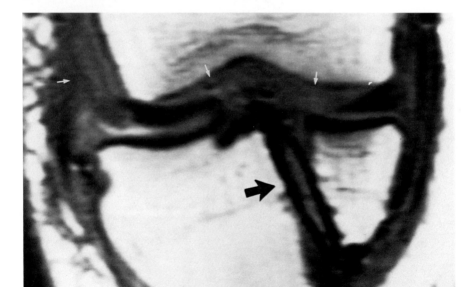

B

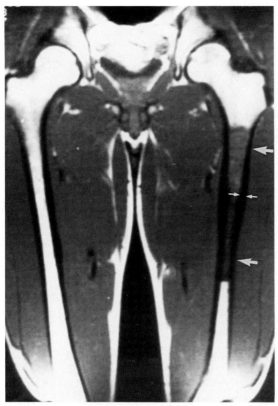

FIG. 6.68. Coronal (**A**, 800/20) and axial (**B**, 1,500/40; **C**, 1,500/80) MR images from a 20-year-old man with a 1-year history of an unhealed stress fracture of the left femur and little callus formation. The coronal MR image reveals an extensive area of decreased signal intensity where the fatty marrow has been replaced (*large arrows*), and there is thickening of the cortex (between *small arrows*). In the axial views, the tissue within the left marrow cavity shows intermediate signal intensity on the balanced image, and higher signal intensity on the T_2-weighted image, much like the signal changes recorded within the testicle (*curved arrow*). At surgery, this entire area was found to have been replaced primarily with a large cystic cavity, although there were cells diagnostic of a Ewing's sarcoma within them. The testicles and the neoplasm probably had the same MRI characteristics because of the high fluid content in each tissue. Tumor (or edema) has invaded the muscles of the left thigh (*straight white arrows,* **C**); the epididymis is also noted (*small arrow*).

A

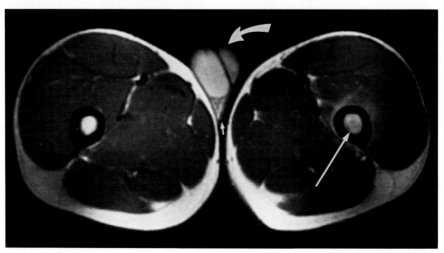

B

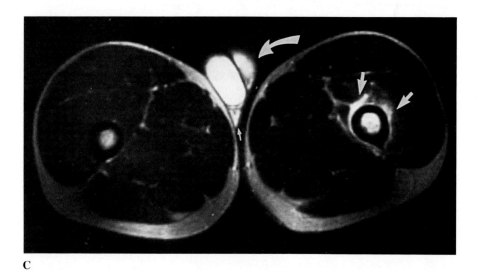

C

FIG. 6.68. continued.

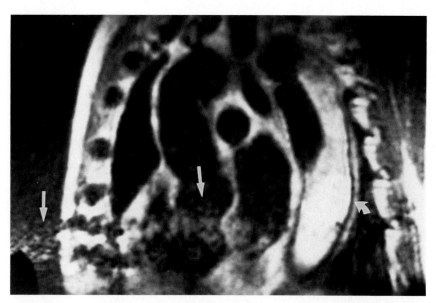

FIG. 6.69. Sagittal MRI study (1,500/25) obtained at 0.34 T with a resistive-magnet system from a patient with a dissection of the descending thoracic aorta (*curved white arrow*). Artifacts due to cardiac pulsations in the phase-encoded-axis direction are noted (*white arrows*).

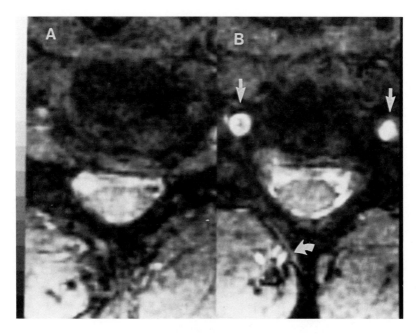

FIG. 6.70. Two axial images (**A,** 1,500/40; **B,** 1,500/80) through the cervical spine in a patient being evaluated for subglottic stenosis reveal even-echo rephasing. Note the even-echo rephasing with increased contrast enhancement in a bull's-eye pattern (*arrows*). There is also some even-echo rephasing occurring in the small veins in the paraspinous muscles (*curved arrow*). Scans were obtained at 1.5 T using a 3-mm slice thickness.

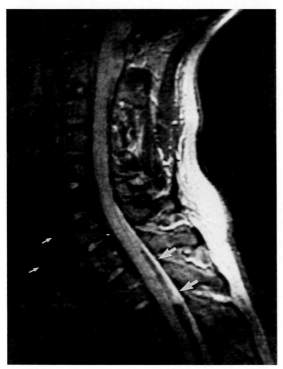

FIG. 6.71. Sagittal MR image (1,500/75) from a normal 6-year-old male revealing multiple pulsation-motion artifacts along the phase-encoded axis (*small white arrows*). CSF pulsation has produced flow voids anterior to the spinal cord, and slow flow or turbulence has produced increased intensity (*large white arrows*) posteriorly. Also note artifactual striations within the cord itself due to the CSF pulsations.

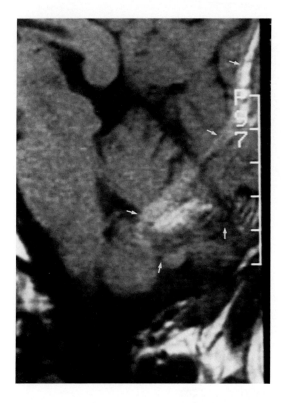

FIG. 6.72. MR image of the brainstem and cerebellum, with a wraparound artifact of the nose and forehead (*arrows*) that has been superimposed over the cerebellum and posterior cerebrum. These artifacts should not be misinterpreted as pathological areas within the brain itself.

Aliasing or Wraparound Artifacts

Fold-around or wraparound artifacts occur when the diameter of the object to be imaged exceeds the field of view of the scanner. Frequency-encoded-axis wraparound artifacts are due to low data-sampling rates. Tissues outside the field of view are reassigned to positions contralateral to their anatomic positions (Fig. 6.72).

Metallic Artifacts

Ferromagnetic clips and other ferromagnetic materials cause distortions in the main magnetic field. The most common appearance of a metallic-clip artifact is signal loss, usually accompanied by a mild degree of distortion. There may also be surrounding or offsetting areas of increased signal intensity (Fig. 6.73).

Chemical-Shift Artifacts

During the readout phase in 2DFT imaging, one dimension of the spatial information is obtained by frequency encoding. In clinical imaging, the Larmor fre-

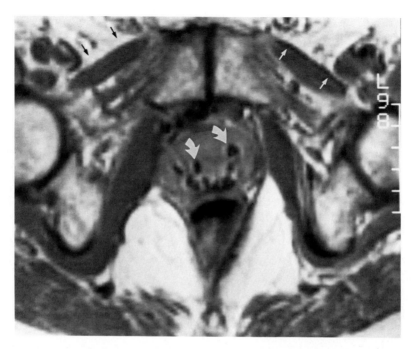

FIG. 6.73. Axial MR image through the pelvis from a patient with known prostatic carcinoma and iridium seeds within the carcinoma. Note the signal loss, accompanied by surrounding increased signal (*curved white arrows*). Metallic artifacts usually are easily recognized and can be identified from careful inspection of the image. However, unusual or unexpected artifacts may occur and can simulate pathological conditions. Some eye makeup that is cobalt-based can also produce metallic artifacts when imaging the orbit. Chemical-shift artifacts due to the fat/water interface around the pectineus muscle anterior to the pubic bones (*small arrows*) are indicated by the band of increased intensity (*black arrows*) on the left of the image and the band of decreased intensity (*white arrows*) on the right.

quency of hydrogen molecules is higher in water than in fat. The difference in the two frequencies is relatively small, but increases with increasing magnetic fields. When the frequency gradient is applied, the molecules in the selective slice increase or decrease their frequency of precession according to their assigned slice-selection frequency. Position is thus linearly related to the gradient field. Because hydrogen molecules in fat are precessing more slowly than those in the surrounding water (e.g., muscle tissue), they will be seen by the scanner as precessing slower than they should for their location. The signal from fat will therefore be assumed to originate from an incorrect location, causing the so-called chemical-shift artifact. Steeper gradients decrease, to some extent, the amount of chemical shift in an image, but at higher B_0 fields this can become a significant problem (Fig. 6.73). Gradient echo sequence shift effects were discussed in the flow imaging section, see Fig. 6.40.

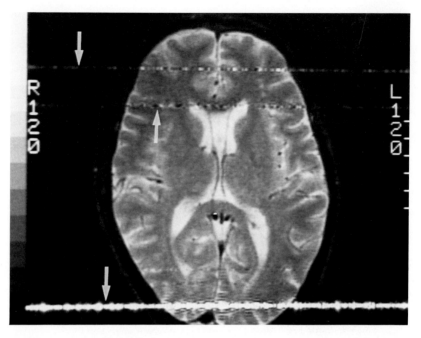

FIG. 6.74. T₂-weighted MR image with significant RF artifact (*arrows*). These artifacts are perpendicular to the frequency-encoded axis, which is oriented vertically in this patient. The RF artifact can be distinguished from the zero-line artifact (see Chapter 8) because a zero-line artifact is parallel with the frequency-encoded axis.

Radio-frequency (B₁) Field Artifacts

If radio-frequency sources in the vicinity of an MRI scanner are in the frequency range of those being used in obtaining the MR images, the RF leak will be seen as an artifact in the image. If it is a wide-band noise containing multiple frequencies, the entire image may be diffusely degraded. More frequently, however, the noise contains a limited range of frequencies or narrow-band noise that appears as "zippers" within the image. The important point in recognizing this type of artifact is that the abnormality is projected perpendicular to the frequency-encoded axis (Fig. 6.74). The exact position of the RF artifact on the image depends on the frequency of interference relative to the central frequency of resonance of the imager being used in the frequency-encoded axis. This artifact should not be confused with the zero-line artifact that always occurs parallel to the frequency-encoded axis (see Chapter 8, Fig. 8.14). In a zero-line artifact, the signal from each point in the selective slice that is normally represented by a sync function (sin x/x) drops off rapidly about a given central point with a series of side lobes. The zero-line artifact, however, appears as a high-amplitude point with very high side lobes of the sync function. The side lobes account for the dark pattern of the artifact in the final image, which is parallel to the frequency-encoded axis.

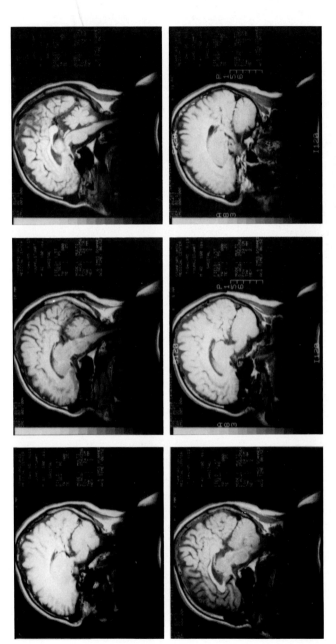

FIG. 6.75. A sequential series of sagittal MRI studies revealing significant intensity differences between slices. This artifact is due to poor slice profiling and the preexcitation sequence used (1.5 T).

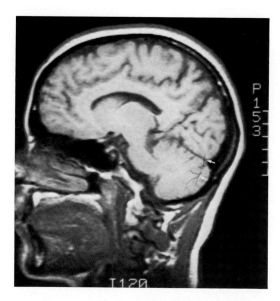

FIG. 6.76. Sagittal MR image with a static-electric-discharge artifact over the cerebellum (*arrows*).

Other MRI Artifacts

Other, less frequently encountered intensity artifacts can occur because of poor slice profile related to inhomogeneous gradients and/or RF or because of preexcitation techniques introduced by the manufacturer (Fig. 6.75). Static electrical discharges usually are fairly easily identified (Fig. 6.76). An artifact characteristic of radial scanning, in which images are obtained in a circular pattern around a fixed point, appears as a long, low-intensity curvilinear stripe where slices overlap (Fig. 6.77). Another artifact occurs in inversion-recovery images and is known as the bounce-point artifact (Fig. 6.47E). As previously discussed, inversion-recovery imaging consists of a 180° pulse followed by a 90° pulse. In magnitude-sensitive reconstruction, the absolute value of the MR signal is reflected in the image. Following a 180° pulse, however, T_1 relaxation occurs and passes through a null point on the x axis that usually is equal to 69% of the T_1 value of the tissue. Bounce-point artifacts may simulate air or calcifications in structures of mixed T_1 relaxation times. The artifacts may produce interface enhancements, such as between gray and white matter, or the fat/water interfaces in other parts of the body. Illustrations of these and other artifacts are indicated throughout this book, and many illustrations are discussed in other chapters on contrast and flow imaging.

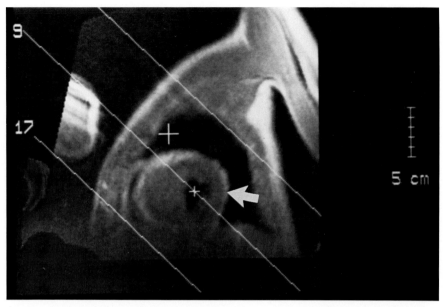

A

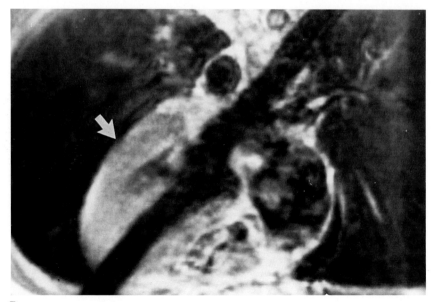

B

FIG. 6.77. A sagittal MRI localizer view (**A**) and an axial image from a radial sequence demonstrating the radial artifact as a low-intensity curvilinear stripe through the image. The patient has myocardiopathy, with generalized enlargement of the myocardium (*white arrow*). The imaging sequence was obtained around a point in the left ventricle indicated by the cross-hair (**A**). The artifact in **B** occurs where the radial slices overlap in scanning through the rotation point in the cavity of the left ventricle (0.34 T resistive magnet).

Chapter 7

Practicing MRI in a Changing Economic Environment

It is better to be a turtle with a compass than a rabbit with a map, at times. At least that was the message of a *Harvard Business Review* article by Robert H. Hayse in November 1985 recommending a strategy for dealing with situations marked by uncertainty and change. If there is one message that has come through loudly and clearly to everyone involved with MRI and MR spectroscopy, it is the message of change. Technical developments and applications in MRI are undergoing a bewildering rate of change, and acquisition of these high-priced MRI scanners is coming into direct conflict with broad cost-containment efforts. This is a new factor making the purchase and use of these hi-tech big-ticket items considerably riskier than would have been the case in a time of cost reimbursement. During stable periods, such as the cost-reimbursement environment of the recent past, microeconomic issues are most important. The certainty of such an environment facilitates detailed, long-range planning, and cost reimbursement can be relied on to cover a lot of sins of inefficiency. During uncertain periods, early intelligence about macroeconomic changes is critical, and planning is best served by plotting a general course and making incremental decisions. We are certainly in such a period today in the health-care industry in this country. Magnifying the impact of these changes is the fact that health care is the third largest business in the United States, behind food and housing, and market forces previously have never been very important in health-care delivery.

There was a joke common among the MBA candidates in my class at the Stanford Graduate School of Business: "A doctor making a bad business decision is redundant." In some cases that is true, but this is a below-the-line observation about investments purchased out of disposable income. The critical difference now is that bad business decisions involving the practice of medicine certainly will adversely impact physicians' incomes. An important distinction to be made in undertaking an economic analysis of MRI concerns the differential impacts of the various macro-economic factors on the professional fees charged for interpreting the examinations, as opposed to the technical fees charged in conjunction with operation of the scanners themselves. Any individual attempting to make a decision about entering the field of MRI should consider setting up a practice specifically designed to interpret

MRI studies for referring physicians, quite apart from the decision whether to own, lease, or not be involved with the technical operation of the scanner and the scanning facility.

The most important macroeconomic changes affecting the practice of MRI have been changes in health-care financing. In order to understand these changes, it is important to review the past history of health-care expenditures. In 1966, prior to the broad development of the Medicare program and the Great Society initiatives, the federal government was paying approximately 13% of health-care costs, and total expenditures were $41.1 billion. By 1981, the government portion had risen to 29%, with $255 billion total expenditures. However, if the past was frightening, the future looked terminal. An extrapolation to 1990 indicated a total expenditure of $685 billion, with the government assuming approximately a 40% share of those expenditures. Corporations, too, are beginning to worry about these expenditures. Many large corporations, even those in the business of producing big-ticket imaging systems, have health-care benefits as one of their major line-item budget expenditures. The response from both government and private industry has been to find ways to reduce the demand for services and to reduce the utilization of health-care services. This has taken the form of diagnostic related groups (DRGs) for hospital-based patients and prepaid or capitated arrangements for other types of health care. Current projections indicate that, nationally, 65% of the population will be covered by PPOs or HMOs by 1990, with HMOs covering approximately 20% of total health-care delivery. Decreased demand for health services, in the form of discounted fee structures, and closer attention by third-party payors to utilization, is one of the factors that increase the risk in practicing MRI in this changing economic environment.

Physician and patient demographics are other factors that are drastically changing. According to the Graduate Medical Education National Advisory Committee (GMENAC), there will be a 30% excess of physicians by 1990 (Table 7.1). That study is projecting an excess of 63,000 physicians, overall, by 1990. Within the area of diagnostic radiology, projections indicate a nearly saturated situation, with the supply of radiologists increasing by approximately 4% per year. The excess of physicians undoubtedly will further exacerbate the struggles already occurring between the cognitive- and procedure-oriented physicians. The results of these struggles could have considerable impact on the professional fee structure currently associated with the interpretation of MR images. The demographic shift within the country is another important factor bearing on MRI practice. The Census Bureau reported for the 1980–1985 period that Florida, California, Texas, and Arizona were the top gainers in population, whereas Michigan, Ohio, Illinois, New York, and Pennsylvania were the biggest losers of population in that period.

Other trends under the general rubric of "unbundling the medical monopoly" represent efforts to allow non-M.D. professionals to compete with M.D.s in providing of medical services. Nurse practitioners, physician's assistants, and osteopaths are generally gaining credentials in this area throughout the country. Dental hygienists are attempting to be licensed to practice without a dentist's supervision. Recently, in Florida, pharmacists won the right to prescribe a limited number of

TABLE 7.1. *GMENAC projections for 1990*

Physician category	Needed	Available	Excess
M.D.s	473,000	536,000	63,000
Radiology[a]			
D_x[b]	20,165	20,086	(79)
R_x[c]	2,513	2,506	(7)

[a]Openings: military, VA, academic.
[b]790 diplomates/year.
[c]95 diplomates/year.

drugs directly to patients without the necessity of obtaining a physician's prescription.

Finally, it is important to bear in mind what is happening to the physician population in medical centers and research-oriented institutions. Although the recent impact of budget projections for NIH research funding did not look too bad, closer scrutiny revealed that the majority of the research funds were being taken up by defense-oriented research on "Star Wars" and other military programs. Biological research through 1987 has remained relatively flat in constant dollars. But if these trends are projected forward, there could be considerable cutbacks in the overall research monies available, and this would further drive physicians out of the research institutions around the country, making more available for private practice of radiology and MRI positions. Further exacerbating these trends is the general oversupply of hospital beds in this country. According to an estimate by one New York consulting firm, 200,000 beds (or approximately 20% of capacity) will be converted to other purposes or closed outright by 1990. This reduction in the number of hospitals open for business in this country could severely impact physicians who have a traditional hospital base, such as radiologists, anesthesiologists, and pathologists; RAPs, as they are called, are already being subjected to attempts to include their fees under the DRG prospective-payment system.

Microeconomic analysis of these macroeconomic trends suggests falling prices for both professional and technical medical and MRI services. If the demand for physician services decreases both in terms of payments and in terms of units of utilization, the overall prices paid for those services must certainly decrease. If, at the same time, the numbers of physicians available to provide services are increasing and other non-M.D. professionals are taking over more of the health-care-delivery program, this is bound to put further pressure on professional and technical fees (Fig. 7.1).

Evidence that these forces are already being felt is the increasing attention physicians are paying to their own personal financial management. The increasing popularity of journals such as *Medical Economics* (P.O. 55, Oradell, New Jersey 07649), and the success of physician's financial advisory services such as the *DR_x Investor* (P.O. 4824, Stanford, California 94305) is specific evidence of this trend.

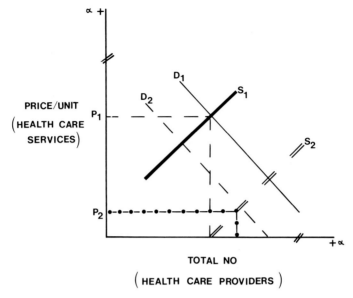

PRICE/UNIT
$\left(\begin{array}{c}\text{HEALTH CARE}\\\text{SERVICES}\end{array}\right)$

TOTAL NO

$\left(\text{HEALTH CARE PROVIDERS}\right)$

FIG. 7.1. Schematic supply–demand curves illustrate the effect of falling unit demand for health-care services and increasing supply of health-care providers. Assuming unit pricing structure (P_1) in the cost-reimbursement environment, as HMO and PPO programs place downward pressure on utilization and obtain discounted prices for health-care services, the demand schedule falls from D_1 to D_2. If the number of health-care providers increases at the same time, the supply schedule shifts from S_1 to S_2. The result is a certain fall in the price paid per unit of health care (P_2). These changes are equally applicable to professional fees and technical fees in interpreting and obtaining MRI studies.

Buying expensive $2 million MRI scanners in this environment cannot be taken lightly.

During this period of uncertainty, physicians need to learn to utilize new techniques to serve as a "compass" to guide them through this changing and treacherous environment. One important question must be asked before initiating an MRI service: Who are my clients? The list of possibilities includes the following:

Referring Physicians
Hospitals
Third Parties
Patients

For most specialist physicians, referrals from primary-care physicians have provided the most important relationship. Hospital-based physicians such as radiologists, pathologists, and anesthesiologists may also find a considerable part of their business related to direct patient visits to hospitals. For most physicians, at this time, the answer to "Who are my clients?" will include a mix of referring primary physicians and hospitals. But the pattern is evolving toward third-party payors packaging PPOs and HMOs to serve the interest of patients. Powerful forces are at work driving this transition.

Prior to the 1980s, the federal government had pursued a program of central planning to solve the health-care problems in the United States. In a regulated, politically controlled environment, the lobbyists and political action committees are the influential groups controlling resource allocation. However, in the current environment, some market forces are being brought to bear on the problem of rising health-care costs. Free markets generally are a good deal for the consumer, and consumers also become the powerful and influential group in allocating resources. The losers are the politicians and the lobbyists. This is why many establishments love regulation and consequent influence over taxing policy. It is a way to keep subsidies flowing, to keep competitors from entering the field, and to reduce the power of the consumer. And regulation gives politicians an excuse for doing something. In health care, there is no doubt that conflicts between patients (or consumers of health-care services who want high-quality care) and corporations and governmental units (who basically are focused on decreasing health-care costs) will occur, but patients, represented by their third-party payors, are likely to become the referral source for people practicing MRI at some point in the future.

Environment	*Influential Group*
Regulated	Lobbyists
Free market	Consumers

As patients' (consumers') preferences become more important in health-care economics, techniques for ascertaining their preferences also become more important. Two marketing research tools—conjoint analysis and trade-off analysis—are designed not only to identify the factors that are important to customers but also to assign a relative value (or utility weighting) to each of those factors. For example, in a study we recently performed for a multispecialty medical group, both referring physicians and patients identified short waiting times and rapid turnaround of MRI reports as being important. However, trade-off and conjoint analysis revealed that patient waiting time was not particularly important to referring physicians, whereas having the results of the MRI study and, if possible, even the hard copy prior to the patient's next visit was extremely important. However, for patients, waiting time at the MRI facility was considerably more important than how quickly the report was issued. The concept is to be certain that those parts of the MRI facility's operation that are valued by the users of that facility are kept in the best and most efficient operating order. Spending a considerable amount of time building efficiencies into a part of the MRI facility that are not valued particularly by the clients or customers of that facility can be a waste of resources.

Strategic planning is another technique that has not been used by physicians in the past, but is becoming more important, specifically, the portion of strategic planning dealing with the strategic business unit (SBU). A SBU (Fig. 7.2) can be defined as any subdivision or activity within the organization. The three important components of SBU analysis are to identify the number of full-time-equivalents (FTE) involved in the activity, to define a measure of value, and to define a historical measure of growth. As shown in the SBU figure, the desired position is to achieve a high value and high rate of growth provided by a small number of FTEs. Conversely, the worst position is to have a large number of individuals involved in an activity with low value and declining volume.

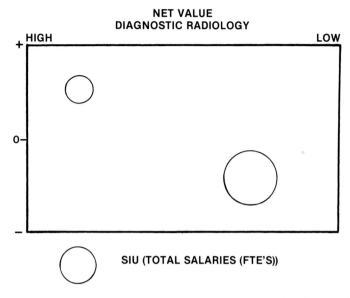

FIG. 7.2. The SBU can be defined as any subdivision or activity within the organization. In imaging, we have redefined them as SIUs. The three important components of SBU analysis are the number of FTEs involved in the activity (illustrated by the sizes of the circles in these diagrams), a defined measure of value (defined as revenue in these diagrams), and a historical measure of growth (defined as examinations, e.g., chest X-ray, CT scan, or MR image). The desired position is to have a high value and high growth provided by a small number of FTEs. Conversely, the worst position is to have a large number of individuals involved in an activity with low value and declining volume.

We have applied this type of analysis to both large medical clinics and medical centers. We have defined the SBU as a strategic imaging unit (SIU) for purposes of this analysis and have taken as the measure of volume the number of units of any particular examination under consideration. The unit of value is the net revenue per FTE performing that activity. Figures 7.3 and 7.4 illustrate this type of analysis by modality. The SIUs with high-volume growth are MRI, mammography, and ultrasound in this particular medical clinic. Of some concern is the fact that angiography is a very high producer of revenue per FTE, but its volume is declining sharply. Application of this type of analysis specifically to the group's MRI operation is shown in Fig. 7.5. The SIUs used here were the MR images from patients with neurological, bone, oncologic (CA), pediatric, and cardiovascular problems. At the time of this analysis, the neurological studies were in a phase of high growth, generating high net revenue. The major strategic decision generated by this type of analysis was in the recognition that the volume of chest and abdomen studies was increasing, but revenues were not, because of lack of reimbursement. Considerable effort subsequently was expanded in obtaining reimbursement for these studies in an effort to move this SIU toward the upper-left-hand corner. Generally speaking, resources should be deployed toward SIUs with high growth rates. And an alarm

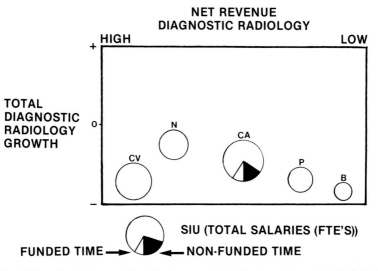

FIG. 7.3. SIU analysis by modality. We have applied this type of analysis to both large medical clinics and medical practitioners. We have defined the SBU as an SIU for purposes of this analysis and taken as the measure of volume the number of units of any particular examination under consideration. The unit of value is the net revenue per FTE performing that activity. The diagrams are working diagrams used in the analysis of this group. Time spent not performing studies was accounted for according to whether it was funded (e.g., paid expert witness) or nonfunded (e.g., vacation). Of some concern is the fact that the cardiovascular SIU is a very high revenue producer per FTE, but its volume is declining sharply. Illustrated are cardiovascular (CV), neuroradiology (N), oncology (CA), pediatrics (P), and bone (B).

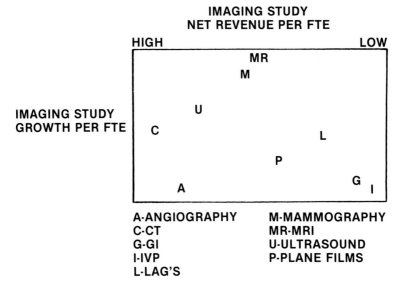

FIG. 7.4. An analysis of the same group as in Fig. 7.3 broken down by modality and net revenue per FTE. MRI mammography and ultrasound are in desirable positions for this group, and angiography is again in a worrisome position.

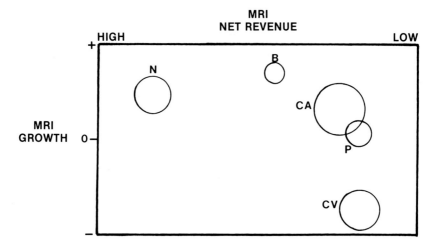

FIG. 7.5. SIU analysis of the group's MRI operations. The SIUs used here were the MR images performed in the various cases: neurological, bone, oncologic, pediatric, and cardio-vascular. At the time of this analysis, the neurological studies were in a phase of high growth, generating high net revenue. The major strategic decision generated by this type of analysis involved the recognition that the volume of chest and abdomen studies was increasing, but revenues were not, because of lack of reimbursement. Considerable effort subsequently was expended to obtain reimbursement for these studies in an effort to move this SIU toward the upper-left-hand corner. Resources should be deployed towrad SIUs with high growth rates. An alarm should go off when a high-revenue-generating SIU begins to experience a volume decline (as illustrated by CV in Fig. 7.3).

should be set off when a high-revenue-generating SIU begins to experience a decline in volume.

The foregoing discussion has dealt mainly with issues normally not emphasized in the usual consideration of acquisition of MRI scanning equipment. This type of analysis usually focuses on the various cost and revenue factors intrinsically related to the MRI scanner itself. A typical check list of factors generally provided by the equipment manufacturers is shown in Table 7.2.

This type of analysis is available from virtually every manufacturer of MRI equipment, and one fairly easy way to get an expert analysis of one manufacturer's assumptions and spread-sheet setup is to turn it over to a second manufacturer for comment. One important factor to understand in evaluating the projections one is given is the discounted cash flow, or net present-value analysis, which accounts for the time value of money in ways that a simple break-even analysis does not.

THE TIME VALUE OF MONEY

Among all of the alternatives offered by manufacturers, which should one choose? The two principles are simple: (1) Time and money are interchangeable. (2) The merits of all investments must be adjusted for risk. The most important concept in ranking the relative merits of investments is the *time value of money*.

TABLE 7.2. *Economic parameters*

System price	$2,035,000
Site cost	$600,000
Supply cost per procedure	$20
Maintenance (annually)	$135,000
Cryogen contract/service	$65,000
Personnel	$80,000
Power rate per kilowatt-hour	0.067
Overhead	$60,000
Annual days of operation	260
Bad debt/contractual allowances	15%
Technical fee	$550
MRI volume:	
Year 1	2,080 (40 patients/week)
After year 1	3,120 (60 patients/week)
Income tax	38%
Sales tax	5%
System lease	9.5% for 5 years
Site-purchase amortization	15% over 25 years
Investment tax credit	None
Profit (measured in terms of net cash flow, with consideration of time value of money)	12%

Source: General Electric Co.

Time and money are interrelated, and, in general, time is a more important factor than money. What we are trying to do is relate two sums of money with respect to the time interval between them. In other words, if we presently have a certain amount of money and designate that as P, and at some point in the future we shall have another amount of money and designate that AF, we can pictorially represent this relationship as follows:

$$P \qquad \ldots AF$$
$$0 \quad 1 \quad 2 \quad 3 \ldots N$$

P equals nominal dollars held presently. AF equals nominal dollars at some point in the future. N equals the number of time units elapsed between the two sums. The values computed for $1.00 placed in an account yielding 10% per year are shown on a time scale similar to that used earlier:

$$
\begin{array}{lcccccc}
\text{year} & 0 & 1 & 2 & 3 & \ldots & 10 \\
\$ & & 1 & 1.10 & 1.20 & 1.331 \ldots & 2.594
\end{array}
$$

The values shown are *time-related equivalent amounts*. In other words, if the expected return is 10%, then $1.00 now is equal to $1.10 in 1 year, or $2.549 after 10 years. If we turn our dollar over to a bank now, it is all the same whether it gives us $1.10 in 1 year or $2.594 in 10 years and will make no difference to us at the compounding rate of 10%.

Similarly, but perhaps more important, if someone with another investment scheme, such as an investment in an MRI facility, offers to take $1 million from us now and in 10 years pay us $2 million, although that is a 100% profit, it falls far short of our objective if our objective is to make 10% compounded on our money per year. Thus, we can work this equivalent time scale backward and forward and use it to more expertly rank the relative merits of alternative investment opportunities. The interest rate is called the cost of capital, and it and the assumptions made by the company working up the numbers for us are critical. A 20% cost of capital means that the payoff needs to be proportionally greater. A reasonable assumption is to take the projected inflation rate over the expected life of the scanner and run the numbers based on this figure.

Of course, we do not always invest exactly at 10%, and to allow for other interest rates or rates of return, we can completely. The general equation used in evaluating the discounted cash flow of an investment is as follows:

$$AF_N = P(1 + i)^N$$

where N is years, i is the interest rate, or cost of capital, AF is future dollars, or net cash flow, and P is present value (present value should exceed the scanner's cost, i.e., the net present value should be positive).

ASSESSING RISK

Because risk is relative, we must have some standard by which to judge the returns on any given investment. This is best done by using the equation for the present value of a future investment, as we did earlier in this chapter. Once we have analyzed the value of the investment's return, we need a yardstick against which to compare. The place to start is with the truly risk-free investment.

In this country, the closest we can get to a risk-free investment is the 90-day United States Treasury Bill. The United States Treasury has never defaulted and, unless the country completely collapses, will never default on paying the interest on its obligations. (If the government ever defaults, it will not make much difference which investment vehicle we own.) The reason for this, of course, is that the government can always print money to pay its bills, and it must, at all costs, maintain public confidence by paying its debts. We can consider the risk on a 90-day United States Treasury Bill as essentially zero, and everything else will involve some greater degree of risk. Consequently, any other investment we undertake should give us a higher rate of return than the current United States Treasury Bill. In general, the longer the duration, the more uncertainty, and the less liquid the investment, the greater the risk. These factors all must be considered in an investment decision regarding a $1 or $2 million MRI scanner. High-quality MRI using a mobile, leased unit is one way to decrease the time and capital risks in MRI (Fig. 7.6).

The usual conclusion drawn after a discounted-cash-flow analysis is that patient volume is critical to the success of an MRI facility. This subject is discussed at length in almost every publication on the economics of MRI and will not be reviewed here. However, there are two points not usually emphasized in the majority

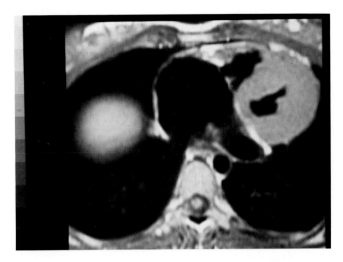

FIG. 7.6. Axial respiratory-compensated cardiac-gated high-quality MR image (TR/TE 779/25) from a mobile 1.5-T system; the patient was a 28-year-old woman with subaortic stenosis and a hypertrophied left ventricle. (Courtesy of the General Electric Co.)

of patient-volume analyses. First, most studies of patient throughput have dealt with issues of pulsing sequence, utilization of multislice fast imaging, or other throughput strategies. A study conducted at Stanford, however, revealed that 53% of a local MRI facility's time is spent on nonscanning activities. It is true that data acquisition takes 42.7% of the total study time, but the majority of total operating time is related to nonscanning activities. Machine downtime and personnel training and practice with the MRI scanner can also adversely affect patient throughput, especially during the first few years of operation. In negotiating with equipment manufacturers, the training and nonscanning operational activities often are neglected. An arrangement whereby the on-site training program is conducted and then followed up by one, two, or three "refresher" on-site programs can eliminate many of these difficulties. There are some MRI facilities operating today that have gone to a 24-hr workday, and they have found that some patients, at least, are willing to fill up these graveyard-shift slots.

Inadequate image quality can also have an adverse impact on referrals and, to some extent, patient throughput. Basic standards of image quality should be a part of every contract negotiation. The best way to assure satisfaction on both sides of this agreement is to find an operating MRI system that produces images of acceptable quality and obtain a tape of some head and body images from that system to establish the appropriate standard. Then images produced by the MRI system being considered for purchase can be compared with that standard.

A break-even analysis often is used in evaluating the financial operation of MRI equipment (Fig. 7.7). The break-even point is taken as the point at which the line describing marginal revenue minus marginal cost crosses the line describing the

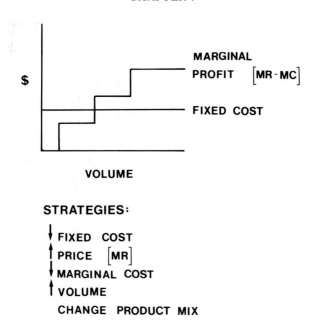

FIG. 7.7. Break-even analysis. Steps indicate incremental scan revenues on the margin. (MR, marginal revenue; MC, marginal cost.)

fixed costs of the center. This line often is presented as a sloping straight line; however, a more accurate way to depict this analysis is, as indicated in the figure, a series of steps—each step representing an incremental scan. Seen in this light, the question of profitability has more to it than just the matter of simple patient through-put. Often, financial success of such an enterprise depends on orchestrating, to best advantage, all components of the system's operations. In this regard, the options available to the site manager include decreasing the initial and total fixed costs, decreasing the marginal costs (those that are incurred each time a scan is per-formed), raising the price per scan, and changing the product mix, in addition to the possibility of increasing patient throughput. The decision whether or not to change the product mix (i.e., the scanning services provided by the MRI center) is facilitated by the SIU analysis presented earlier in this chapter. Generally, resources and marketing efforts should reinforce those SIUs that are experiencing an increase in unit volume and have a relatively high price per FTE. In addition to the possi-bility of operating the MRI unit 24 hr per day, there are other possible choices involving product mix and volume that enter into considerations of strategic plan-ning. MRI has a considerable number of industrial applications. MRI has been used in analyzing core samples from oil fields undergoing tertiary recovery procedures (Fig. 7.8). MRI analysis of water and nutrient uptake in plants is playing an in-creasingly more important role in developing higher-yielding agricultural products (Fig. 7.9). Some centers in Europe have joint-ventured with forest-product com-panies in using CT and MRI scanners, which are effective in evaluating tree growth.

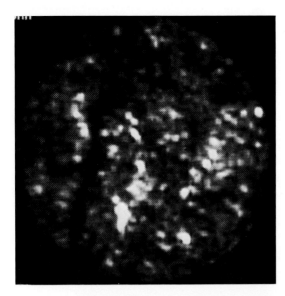

FIG. 7.8. MRI study of a core sample for a petroleum economic model and tertiary-recovery study. The porosity of the core (holes are white in the dolomite core) and measurements of the ability of various detergents and steam to remove hydrocarbons are important findings in these studies. (Courtesy of GE NMR instruments. Fremont, Calif.)

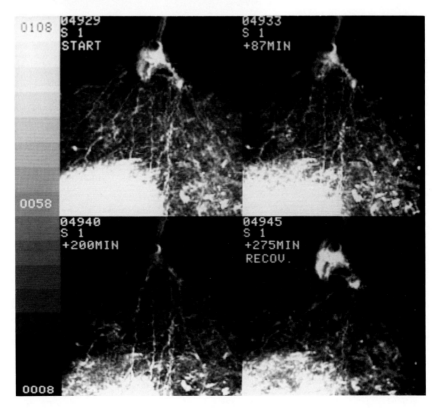

FIG. 7.9. A series of MR images from a plant-root/soil system demonstrating uptake of water (white) from the soil into the root system. Exposure to light stress shows water leaving the cotyledonary area after 87 and 200 min and a recovery at 275 min. (Courtesy of P. A. Bottomley, GE Corporate Research and Development Center, Schenectady, N.Y.)

MRI also is used for evaluating curing rates in resins and plastics and detecting bubbles and predicting burn rates in solid-rock fuels. Two large West Coast aerospace manufacturers use CT scanners and are considering industrial MRI. Depending on the proximity of various types of industries in the area in which an MRI facility is located, late-night industrial services can be provided at a relatively low marginal cost to facilitate the overall economic performance of the MRI facility. These types of alternatives can remove some of the risk in making the MRI decision. Local coils and bird-cage coils are facilitating excellent-quality MRI microscopy and images of domestic and research animals. Off-hour research and educational services for both practicing physicians and residents and fellows may also provide additional opportunities for revenue generation by an MRI center.

Chapter 8

Horizons in MRI and MRS

The horizons in MRI and MR spectroscopy (MRS) are expanding rapidly as new clinical applications are being developed. Paramagnetic contrast media offer the promise of organ-specific changes in proton relaxation. Imaging and spectra using ^{19}F, ^{13}C, ^{23}Na, and ^{31}P are being tested in preliminary clinical applications. Suppression of water and fat is expanding the use of proton data in metabolite evaluation. The ability to obtain localized spectra and image biochemical processes offers great potential for detecting human disease at the early stages of biochemical alteration. Promising MRI and MRS applications that are on the horizon are reviewed briefly in this section.

MRI CONTRAST AGENTS

Intravenously or orally administered paramagnetic, supermagnetic, and ferromagnetic contrast media are rapidly being developed. The first agents used have acted throughout the extracellular space, similar to the way iodinated water-soluble contrast agents have been used in CT scanning. However, agents that are targetable to a specific disease process or organ system are able to detect early cellular dysfunction (Figs. 8.1 and 8.2). Paramagnetic agents have been found to be useful in detecting early breakdown of the blood-brain barrier, including parenchymal lesions of the brain (Fig. 8.3), and abnormal accumulation of contrast agents in the vitreous humor of the eye, and hepatocyte toxicity.

MRI AND MRS WITH MULTIPLE NUCLEAR SPECIES

Other nuclei are potentially useful in MRI. To be useful in MRI, nuclei should be biologically prevalent and also magnetic. For example, although ^{12}C is prevalent

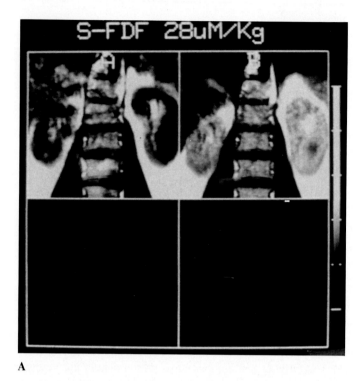

A

FIG. 8.1. **A:** These images before and after infusion of contrast agent were taken from a phase-2 clinical trial. **Left:** Pre-contrast coronal renal image shows good renal outline within the retroperitoneal fat. **Right:** Following intravenous infusion of a paramagnetic contrast agent (S-FDF), a proprietary formulation of ferrioxamine, a nephrogram effect is seen. Also seen are benign cysts within the left renal parenchyma. (Courtesy of Salutar Inc.)

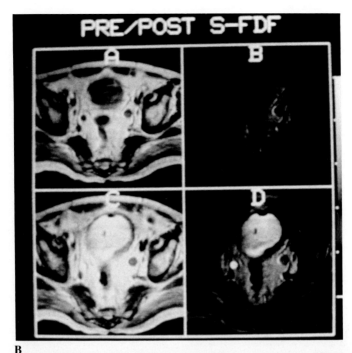

B

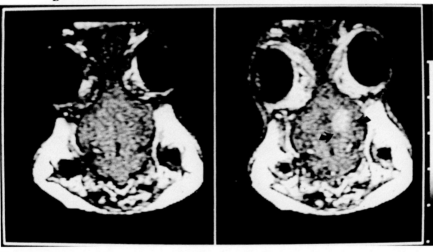

C

FIG. 8.1. *(continued)* **B:** Transaxial images of the pelvis from a patient in a phase-2 clinical trial. Panels A and B (pre-contrast) are the first (25 msec) and second (50 msec) echoes of a standard spin-echo sequence (TR = 600 msec) on a clinical MR imager (1.5 T). The bladder, bilateral hydroureters, and rectum are well seen before contrast injection. Panels C and D (post-contrast) are the same anatomic sections 30 min after S-FDF infusion. In panel D, the left-ureter obstruction and lack of urine flow (low intensity vs. high intensity of contralateral hydroureter) are especially well documented. (Courtesy of Salutar Inc.) **C:** Pre-contrast image of a defect in the blood-brain barrier in rabbit. The left-hand image (spin-echo; TR = 150 msec, TE = 20 msec; 1.5 T) is a transaxial image through the eyes showing a traumatically induced defect in the blood-brain barrier. The image on the right was obtained 30 min following infusion of a paramagnetic contrast agent that does not cross the normal blood-brain barrier. The large central lesion in the left hemisphere is seen only following injection of contrast material *(arrow)*. (Courtesy of Dr. S. Quay, Salutar Inc.)

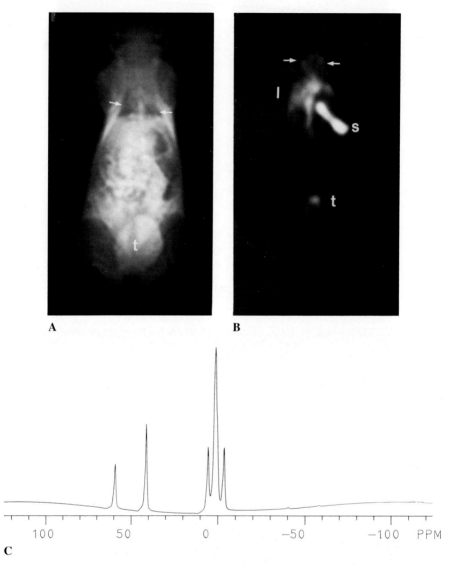

FIG. 8.2. Coronal proton image (**A**) and ¹⁹F image (**B**, 4.7 T CSI scanner) following intra-venous administration of perfluorooctyl bromide (PFOB provided courtesy of Fluoromed Pharmaceutical, Inc.) and (**C**) ¹⁹F spectrum illustrating the four fluorine peaks in PFOB. In obtaining the images shown in **B**, the two upfield peaks were suppressed with an imaging sequence. The images were obtained at 2 T using a projection imaging sequence. Following PFOB administration, the liver (l), spleen (s), and lungs (*arrows*) show high signal intensities due to PFOB within the reticuloendothelial system. Also note some PFOB in the bone marrow of the vertebral column, appearing as a vertical white line between the liver and spleen. PFOB is also taken up in the RIF-1 tumor in this 20-g mouse (t). The lungs appear as low-intensity structures on the proton image (*arrows*).

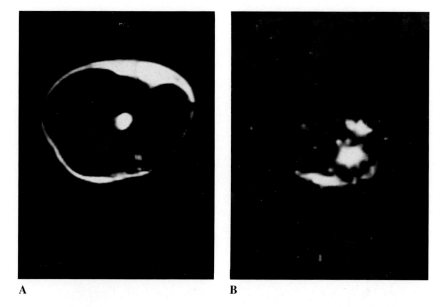

A **B**

FIG. 8.3. Axial fat-proton image (**A**) and ^{13}C image (**B**) of the same section of a human forearm. The image required over 2 hr to obtain, but illustrates the distribution of ^{13}C in the forearm. (Courtesy of Jun Hasegawa, M.S., Asahi Chemical Industry Co., Ltd., Kanagawa, Japan.)

TABLE 8.1. *Properties of nuclei of interest in medicine*

Nucleus	Spin	MHz/T
^{1}H	½	42.6
^{2}H	1	6.5
^{13}C	½	16.7
^{14}N	1	3.1
^{15}N	−½	9.3
^{17}O	−⁵⁄₂	5.8
^{19}F	½	40.1
^{23}Na	³⁄₂	11.3
^{31}P	½	17.2

within the body, it is not magnetic. The isotope ^{13}C is magnetic and potentially useful as an MRI agent, but its biological abundance is only approximately 1%. Thus, the combination of concentration, natural abundance, and the intrinsic relative NMR signal strength establishes the overall NMR signal sensitivity. Table 8.1 lists the nuclei of greatest interest in NMR imaging in medicine in order of decreasing NMR sensitivity.

^{19}F

^{19}F has a resonant frequency closest to that of hydrogen and a very high signal intensity. Little imagable fluorine exists within the body, however, and so any studies involving ^{19}F require biological enrichment. However, there are many agents containing ^{19}F that have predictable biochemical activity within the body and, if traceable through MRI or MRS, offer the possibility of evaluating biochemical processes. Imaging and spectroscopy of the reticuloendothelial system have already been accomplished using perfluorooctyl bromide (PFOB) in animals and humans (Fig. 8.2). ^{19}F MRI and MRS of soluble and emulsified perfluorinated agents have been used in imaging the cardiovascular system, and fluorinated anesthetic agents have been used to estimate brain perfusion and lung ventilation. Fluorine has also been used for evaluating glucose metabolism. Fluorinated emulsions have been used to image carcinomas and detect radiation damage of the lung and liver.

^{13}C

In nature, 99% of carbon occurs as the isotope ^{12}C, which does not have a magnetic moment and therefore does not produce an NMR signal. The remaining 1% is the isotope ^{13}C, which does give a spectrum rich in chemical information. Although ^{13}C NMR is relatively insensitive compared with ^1H or ^{31}P, the possibility of increasing the natural abundance by administering ^{13}C-labeled metabolites may decrease signal acquisition times. Molecules such as fatty acids or glucose can be labeled with ^{13}C, and subsequent NMR chemical analysis can detect the progress of the ^{13}C atom as it is metabolized. The progress of the ^{13}C label follows the metabolic pathways. Because of the low biological concentration of ^{13}C in human tissue, imaging is impractical on a clinical basis; however, some ^{13}C images are beginning to appear from research laboratories (Fig. 8.3).

^{23}Na

^{23}Na is an excellent marker for the extracellular space. In this regard, there have been many attempts to use ^{23}Na in MRI or MRS to detect breakdown in the blood-brain barrier. Extracellular sodium produces an excellent high-intensity signal, as seen in the eye, ventricles, and cisterns of the brain in Fig. 8.4. An interesting adaptation of extracellular-sodium imaging has been developed at the University of New Mexico by R. H. Griffey. Sodium images are obtained before and after intravenous administration of gadolinium. The presence of gadolinium "subtracts out" the sodium from any profused tissues; thus, the post-gadolinium sodium image reveals only sodium that is in a nonperfused space, such as in the center of a large neoplasm (Fig. 8.5).

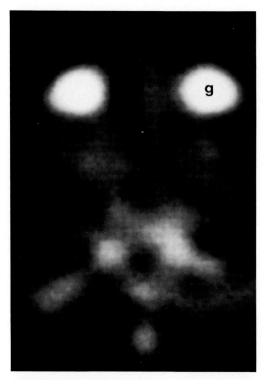

A

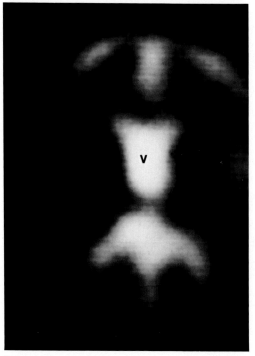

B

FIG. 8.4. ^{23}Na images at the level of the orbits (**A**) and through the lateral ventricles (**B**) illustrating extracellular sodium in the globe of the eye (g) and ventricles (v). High-intensity sodium signal is also seen from the subarachnoid cisterns.

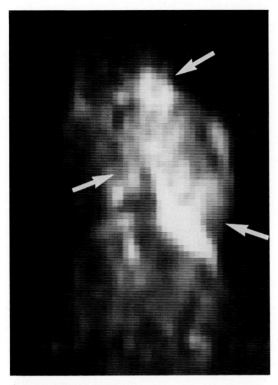

A

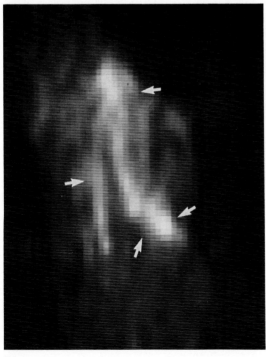

B

FIG. 8.5. Projection ^{23}Na images (4.7 T, CSI 5E scanner) from a mouse with a large tumor before (**A**) and after (**B**) intravenous administration of Gd-DTPA. The sodium image of the tumor (*large arrows,* **A**) is seen to be significantly smaller in the post-Gd study (*arrows,* **B**) because the gadolinium has "subtracted out" sodium in areas where the gadolinium is present. The residual signal represents areas of ischemic or necrotic tumor. (Courtesy of Richard H. Griffey, Ph.D., and Nicholas A. Matwiyoff, Ph.D., and Beatrice Griffey.)

^{31}P

Considerable progress has been made in applying ^{31}P spectroscopy techniques to *in vivo* clinical evaluation. The major challenge for *in vivo* spectroscopy has been accurate localization of voxels from which ^{31}P spectra are sampled. One approach (SLIT DRESS) to this problem has been developed by Bottomley and associates. The slice-selection capability of the scanner is combined with surface-coil localization. This technique has been effective in evaluating muscle, brain, and internal organs such as the heart (Figs. 8.6 and 8.7). Characteristic spectra from these tissues can be resolved on the basis of depth and are easily distinguishable from each other, and interventions such as ischemia and reperfusion are reflected in changes in the ^{31}P spectrum.

Although considerable variations are seen among malignant neoplasms, MRS is becoming very useful for evaluation of cancer patients. Concentrations of phosphomonoesters, inorganic phosphate, and phosphodiesters are elevated in malignant neoplasms, whereas phosphocreatine is reduced. Malignant tumors tend to be relatively acidic, and pH values can be ascertained from the ^{31}P spectrum because the balance of sodium monophosphate and sodium biphosphate causes the inorganic phosphate line to shift down-field (i.e., toward lower precessional frequencies or ppm) as tissues become more acidic. Cancer therapy can also be evaluated using MRS. In general, the phosphocreatine/inorganic-phosphate ratio increases as long as therapy is efficacious. Nearly complete depletion of tumor energy stores (ATP) is seen in isolated tumor specimens following tumor-necrosis-factor infusion or other tumoricidal interventions. These changes occur before any change in tumor volume or any obvious changes discernible at histological evaluation. Partially effective therapy often is reflected in inorganic-phosphate/phosphocreatine ratios or inorganic-phosphate/ATP ratios.

^{1}H

The horizons in proton imaging are equally as exciting as those using other nuclei in MRI and MRS. Computer screening of large proton data bases, microscopic MRI, and rapid scanning techniques in conjunction with respiratory and cardiac gating are developing rapidly. In addition, imaging and spectroscopy of the chemical-shift differences between fat and water are being used for clinical evaluation of patients, and preliminary laboratory results using water-suppressed (and, in some cases, fat-suppressed) proton spectra and images of metabolites such as lactic acid have been successfully obtained and offer the attractive possibility of metabolic monitoring.

FUZZY-CLUSTER ANALYSIS OF PROTON MRI DATA

MRI is a valuable diagnostic tool with much greater sensitivity to abnormal water content of tissue than other imaging modalities. The data are complex, however, and displaying all the data in a gray-scale image is impossible. Current image inter-

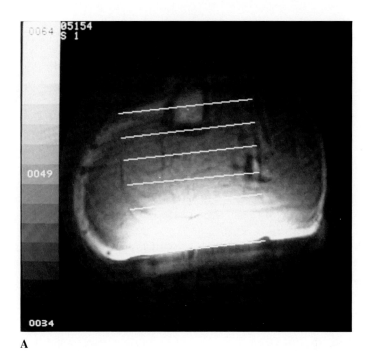

A

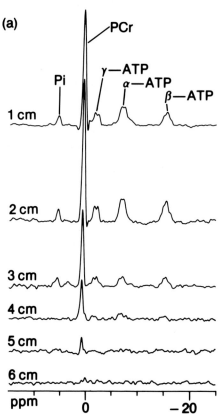

(a)

PCr

Pi

γ—ATP
α—ATP
β—ATP

1 cm

2 cm

3 cm

4 cm

5 cm

6 cm

ppm   0   − 20

B

FIG. 8.6. MRI proton image (**A**) and phosphorus spectra (**B**) from normal calf muscle and MRI proton image (**C**) and ^{31}P spectra (**D**) from normal brain. The ^{31}P spectra were recorded at the indicated depths from the skin-surface coil (1–6 cm). The horizontal white lines indicate the depths at which the ^{31}P spectra were recorded (SLIT DRESS technique). Note the marked differences between the ^{31}P spectra from normal brain and normal muscle. Although the inorganic phosphate is slightly elevated in the top three slices, which may reflect some ischemia in the muscle compressed by the surface coil, the spectra resemble those for normal unsaturated muscle.

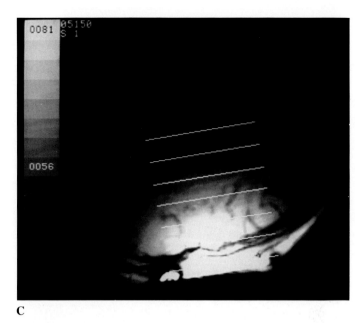

C

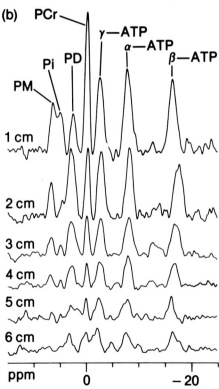

(b)

PCr

γ—ATP

α—ATP

Pi PD β—ATP

PM

1 cm

2 cm

3 cm

4 cm

5 cm

6 cm

ppm   0   −20

D

FIG. 8.6. *(continued)* Spectra from the brain are characterized by phosphomonoester (PM) concentrations that are about half the ATP concentrations at a depth of 2 cm. The phosphodiester (PD) concentrations are approximately comparable to the ATP concentrations. In both spectra, decreases in peak amplitudes with increasing depth correlate with decreased surface-coil sensitivity. This can be seen as a falloff in signal intensity within the proton image. *In vivo* [31]P SLIT DRESS spectra were recorded with the lower leg draped over the surface coil, showing the calf muscle (**A**), and with the head lying sideways on the coil above the left ear (**C**). (PCr) phosphocreatine; (Pi) inorganic phosphate. (Courtesy of P. A. Bottomley, Ph.D., GE R&D Center, Schenectady, N.Y.)

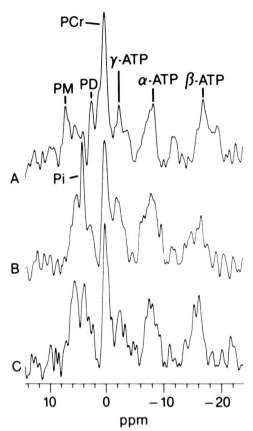

FIG. 8.7. ^{31}P spectra obtained using a localizer technique (SLIT DRESS) recorded from the anterior wall of the left ventricle. The normal-dog-heart ^{31}P spectrum was obtained prior to coronary occlusion (**A**) and demonstrates a normal phosphocreatine/β-ATP ratio. **B:** ^{31}P spectrum acquired following 65 min of coronary occlusion. **C:** Spectrum obtained following reperfusion of the ischemic heart. During coronary occlusion, a marked increased in the inorganic-phosphate peak and a slight down-field shift occurred (**B**). A decrease in inorganic phosphate and marginal restoration of the phosphocreatine/ATP ratio followed coronary reperfusion in the spectrum acquired 100 min following occlusion. (PCr) phosphocreatine; (PD) phosphodiester; (PM) phosphomonoester; (Pi) inorganic phosphate. (Courtesy of P. A. Bottomley, Ph.D.)

pretation requires a semiquantitative "visual synthesis" or "visual cluster analysis" of signal intensities on multiple images based on different MRI parameters. Improved specificity of MRI is likely to come from a more quantitative screening of the data and computerized analysis of multiple MRI factors.

Several computerized image-analysis techniques largely derived from methods developed by NASA for multispectral analysis of LANDSAT satellite images have been applied to MRI. The simplest classification procedure begins with the observer's identification of tissue regions (e.g., tumor, edema, normal, etc.) based on *a priori* knowledge or assumptions about true tissue characteristics. The computer then takes this "supervised" classification scheme and assigns each pixel in the image to the appropriate tissue category. More sophisticated approaches allow "unsupervised" (automated) classification of tissues into categories without observer bias by utilizing the techniques of multivariate statistical analysis.

Fuzzy-cluster analysis is one such technique; it is based on fuzzy mathematical set theory (using partial or "fuzzy" assignment of members to sets). It produces

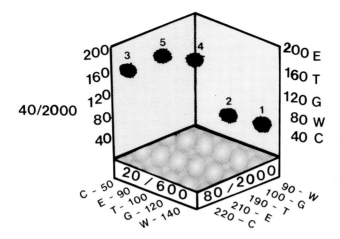

FIG. 8.8. Three-dimensional fuzzy-cluster analysis of the images in Fig. 8.9. A diagrammatic illustration of the distribution of cluster centers representing different tissue types in three-dimensional feature space. The axes of the feature space are formed by the intensity scales of the source T_1-weighted (600/20), T_2-weighted (2,000/80), and intermediate-weighted (2,000/20) images obtained at 1.5 T. The size of each cluster is approximately a radius of 1 standard deviation, with "fuzzy" margins drawn for purposes of illustration: white matter (W and 1), gray matter (G and 2), tumor (T and 4), CSF (C and 3), edema (E and 5).

classified images by fractional assignment (fuzzy membership assignment) of pixels to clusters (tissue classes) based on the Euclidean (geometric) distance of each pixel from the cluster center. The number of source images determines the dimensions of the Euclidean space (feature space) in which the cluster analysis is carried out. Figure 8.8 illustrates a three-dimensional feature space generated by three source images. Any number of source images can be used to generate the classified image. As more qualitatively different source images are used, there is an increased likelihood of separating two tissues with similar signals in one source image on the basis of their signal difference in another source image. The potential for improving tissue specificity beyond that obtainable with visual analysis is great. Preliminary results indicate an improved capacity to uniquely identify cerebral cancer and to distinguish it from surrounding edema (Fig. 8.9). This technique can also be used to precisely assess temporal change (e.g., effectiveness of tumor therapy) and can incorporate image data from other modalities such as CT or position-emission tomography (PET) to form a more comprehensive scheme of tissue classification.

High-resolution MRI and MRS are providing new tools for researchers in basic biological sciences. High-resolution proton imaging of primates is providing a noninvasive technique for evaluating neurological conditions that mimic those found in humans (Fig. 8.10). High-resolution MRI with cardiovascular gating appears to be useful in distinguishing cardiovascular structures as small as those contained in a beating rat heart (Figs. 8.11 and 8.12) or developing embryo (Fig. 8.13).

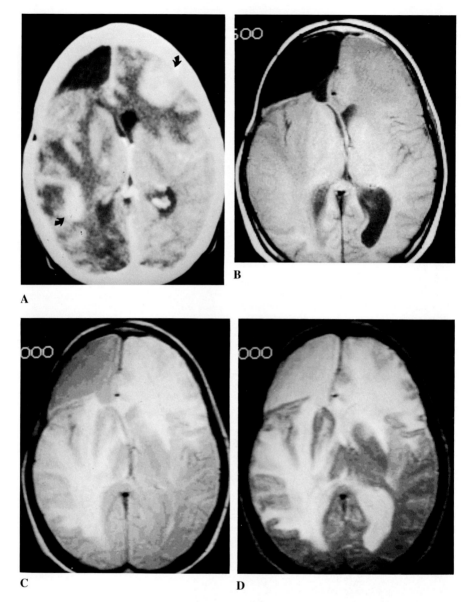

FIG. 8.9. Recurrent astrocytoma. **A:** CT scan showing areas of contrast enhancement in the temporal-lobe and frontal-lobe regions that represent postsurgical recurrence of an astrocytoma (*arrows*). Low-attenuation white-matter edema is seen medially, adjacent to these areas of enhancement. A postsurgical defect filled with CSF is seen in front of the right frontal lobe. **B:** T$_1$-weighted image (TR = 600 msec, TE = 20 msec; 1.5 T) shows minimal contrast between the regions of tumor recurrence and the adjacent lower-signal edema. The regions corresponding to contrast enhancement on the CT scan appear similar to areas of normal brain elsewhere in the image (left temporal and parietal lobes). **C:** The first echo of the spin-echo pulse sequence (TR = 2,000 msec, TE = 40 msec; 1.5 T) shows better contrast than the T$_1$-weighted image between tumor regions and edema. In this image the areas of edema show higher signal than the areas of tumor. However, the regions of tumor still appear similar to normal brain elsewhere in the image. **D:** The second echo of the T$_2$-weighted pulse sequence (TR = 2,000 msec, TE = 80 msec; 1.5 T) shows high contrast between the tumor and the higher-signal edema. However, the tumor regions remain indistinguishable from normal brain in the contralateral hemisphere.

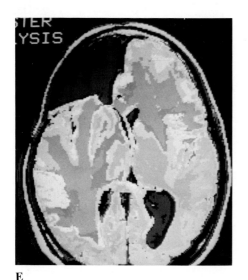

E

FIG. 8.9. *(continued)* **E:** Classified image with tissue categories generated by "unsupervised" fuzzy-cluster analysis. The gray scale is based on the Euclidean distance of each cluster center from the origin of the three axes forming the feature space (the three source-image intensity scales). In this image the contrast between tumor areas and edema is enhanced. More important, the difference between tumor tissue and normal brain elsewhere in the image is clearly depicted. This discrimination is information that cannot be derived by visual inspection of the source images (**B, C,** and **D**). The correspondence of the areas uniquely classified as tumor is very close to the regions of contrast enhancement seen on the CT scan. (Courtesy of R. E. DeLaPaz, M.D.)

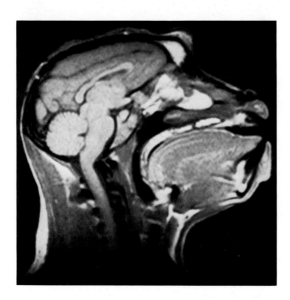

FIG. 8.10. 2-T proton image from normal monkey. Images were collected using the GE CSI spectroscopy imaging system, with automated spin-echo sequence. Image parameters for this sagittal T_1-weighted image were: TR = 400 msec, TE = 15 msec; FOV = 15 cm; slice = 2 mm; NA = 2; matrix = 256 × 256. (Courtesy of R. Hurd, Ph.D., GE NMR Instruments, Fremont, California)

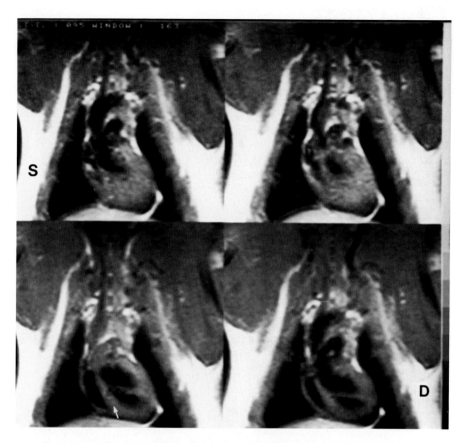

FIG. 8.11. Coronal high-resolution gated right-heart sequence from a 200-g rat demonstrating systole (S) through diastole (D). Note the interventricular septum between the left and right ventricular cavities (*arrow*) and the papillary muscle within the left ventricular cavity. Parameters: CSI 2 T; 3-mm slice; 80 × 80 mm; 128 × 256 raw data, 512 × 512 output; 2 NEX: 2DFT spin-echo; TE = 15 msec, TR = 220–360 msec. The rat heart measures 7 × 10 mm (along long axis). (Courtesy of M. E. Moseley, Ph.D., and W. M. Chew, B.S.)

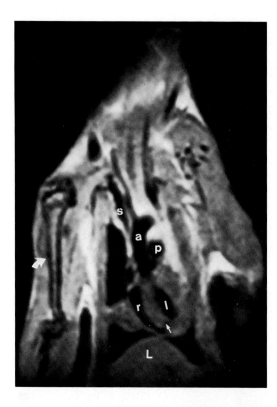

FIG. 8.12. A magnified coronal MRI study from a gated sequence in early diastole: 2 T; CSI; 256 × 256 × 8; 3DFT; FOV = 60 × 60 × 6 mm; output matrix 512 × 512 for each image. Notice the excellent detail in the right forearm bone (*curved arrow*). This is an example of microscopy; pixel size is 280 × 280 × 750 μm (slice); calculated from FOV and raw-data matrix (256 × 256 × 8). Image was gated to the EKG R wave throughout data acquisition. Superior vena cava (s); ascending aorta (a); left main pulmonary artery (p); right ventricular cavity (r); left ventricular cavity (l); interventricular septum (*arrow*); right humerus (*curved white arrow*); liver (L). (Courtesy of M. E. Moseley, Ph.D., and W. M. Chew, B.S.)

FIG. 8.13. MRI of 14-day-old chick egg: 2-mm slice; 100 × 100 mm; 256 × 256; NEX = 4; 2DFT spin-echo; TE = 80 msec, TR = 3,000 msec. Albumen is dark (*large arrow*) with T$_2$ weighting. Eye (bullet) is bright and to the left of the brain (*open arrow*). Spine curves at the bottom of the egg. Knee joint (*short arrow*). (Courtesy of M. E. Moseley, Ph.D., and W. M. Chew, B.S.)

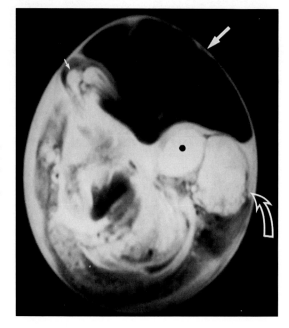

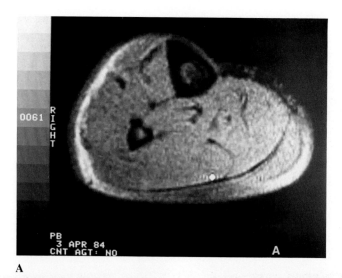

A

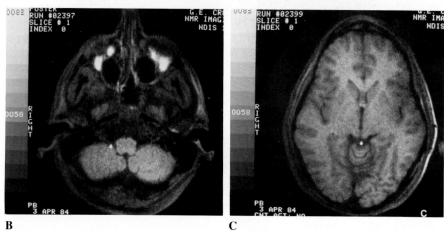

B   C

FIG. 8.14.   MR images of the head and thigh obtained at 1.5 T representing water protons
(**A–C**), conventional MR images (**D–F**) for comparison, and ¹H-CH₂ fat images (**G–I**). The
selective fat and water images were obtained by selective preirradiation of water and CH₂
resonances, respectively. The voxel volume was 1 × 1 × 4 mm; 256 × 256. There is a
central line artifact on each of the images. The central line (*white*) artifact can best be seen
in images **A, D** and **E**.

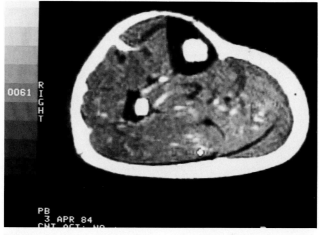

D

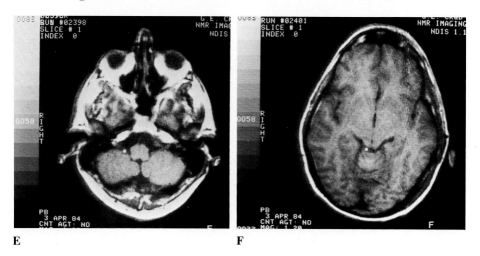

E   F

FIG. 8.14. *(continued)* Images **A, D,** and **G** were obtained through the lower leg; **B, E,** and **H** and **C, F,** and **I** were obtained at the levels of the orbits and lateral ventricles, respectively. (Courtesy of P. A. Bottomley, Ph.D., GE R&D Center, Schenectady, N.Y.)

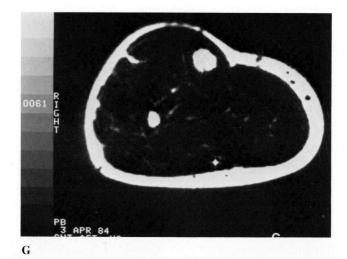

G

H   I

FIG. 8.14. continued.

CHEMICAL-SHIFT MRI AND MRS

The initial experience with chemical shift in clinical imaging presented problems in that the overlapping of different frequencies from water and fat protons appeared to create structures that were not in fact present within the tissue. It was rapidly recognized, however, that discrimination of the chemical environment of a particular nuclear species was practical via spatially localized *in vivo* chemical-shift MRI

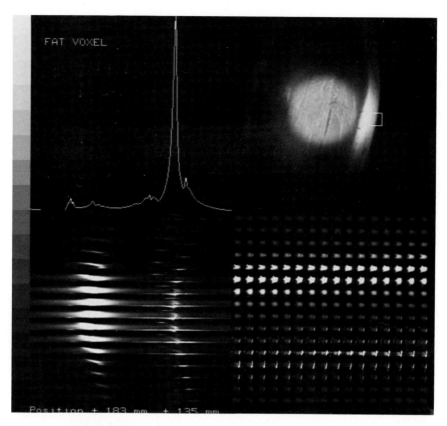

FIG. 8.15. Chemical-shift spectra from normal human gastrocnemius muscle. Upper-right-hand-corner: high-resolution "map" image of human gastrocnemius muscle. Lower-right-hand corner: chemical-shift images showing spatial distribution of water (upper images) and fat (lower images), with frequency resolution of 2 Hz per image and spatial resolution of 1 cm³ per voxel. Lower-left-hand corner: chemical-shift display of spatial images in lower-right-hand corner (chemical-shift vs. spatial-encoding gradient). Upper-left-hand corner: single-voxel spectrum from chemical-shift imaging matrix at position indicated by cursor in "map" image. Spectral bandwidth: 500 Hz with 256 complex points. Note in the fat spectrum resonances from left to right as follows: unsaturated fat, residual water, methylene protons bound to hetero atoms, allgliz hydrogens, "backbone" methylene resonance and terminal methyl resonance. (Courtesy of the General Electric Co.)

and MRS. Recent advances in using higher static magnetic fields, very homogeneous magnets, and steep magnetic-field gradients have enabled the acquisition of images of either fat or water protons within the body. Many techniques of developing chemical-shift images are available; the one presented in this section involves selective radiation of all other species, other than the one desired to be imaged, in the absence of imaging gradients. Thus, the chemical-shift information is selected

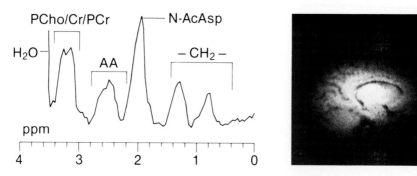

FIG. 8.16. Water- and fat-suppressed proton spectra and metabolite image of human brain. (Courtesy of P. A. Bottomley, Ph.D., GE R&D Center, Schenectady, N.Y.)

prior to the application of conventional MRI or MRS sequences. ^{1}H-H$_2$0 and ^{1}H-CH$_2$ images are obtainable using this technique, with little overlap of the fat-proton signal in the water image (Figs. 8.14 and 8.15). Suppression of the water and fat peaks in the proton spectra has permitted acquisition of spectra and images of localized metabolites (Fig. 8.16). Detection of lactic acid in this manner has been accomplished and may be useful in detecting ischemic tissue in the heart, lung, brain, abscesses, or malignant neoplasms.

Chapter 9

Hazards and Site Planning

Site planning for MRI facilities is becoming less complicated. Electrically shielded magnets, permanent and resistive magnets with small fringe fields, and the prospect of new alloys that will be superconducting at relatively high temperatures are all factors that work to alleviate the problems encountered in establishing MRI centers. Medical diagnosis utilizing NMR scanners may be one of the first diagnostic modalities in which there is more risk for the operator of the equipment than for the patient (Fig. 9.1). To date, no adverse effects attributable to NMR imaging have been reported in patients or volunteers. The major risk to operators of NMR systems comes from the high magnetic fields associated with these devices. Any metallic object that is free to move can become a potentially lethal projectile if it comes into close proximity to these strong magnetic fields. To avoid this problem, the access routes to all imaging units are guarded by metal detectors similar to those used for screening airports and other public places. However, the sensitivity levels for these detectors in NMR imaging units are set extremely low, and many false alarms occur; these alarms often activate spontaneously, and after some time there is a tendency for personnel to begin ignoring these signals. This lack of vigilance has the potential to produce serious consequences. An unexpected risk of Gaussian carditis was reported in the August 12, 1982, issue of the *New England Journal of Medicine*. Another peripheral problem concerns credit cards, which are not metallic and therefore do not activate metal sensors; however, credit cards carrying magnetic codes can be demagnetized and consequently will not work in any system based on the card's magnetic code. To avoid this embarrassment, all metallic objects and all credit cards should be removed from one's person before entering the MRI facility.

One major advantage of NMR imaging systems, as compared with CT scanners, is that patients are not exposed to ionizing radiation. There is no evidence at the moment to suggest that there is a health hazard from the imaging techniques currently used. Nevertheless, patients are exposed to relatively intense static, gradient-induced, and RF-induced magnetic fields, and the possibility of either early or late adverse effects from such exposure must be considered.

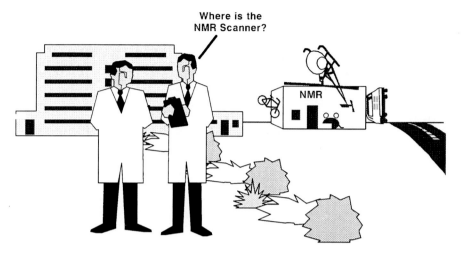

FIG. 9.1.   NMR hazards.

MAGNETIC FIELDS

Most of the data accumulated regarding static magnetic fields have been obtained from animal studies at the 1-T level. Small electrical potentials in the large blood vessels that are generated by the flow of blood perpendicular to the magnetic field have been observed. Theoretically, if the flow potential were sufficiently large, it could affect the heart either by direct stimulation or by indirect stimulation of the pressure receptors situated in the aortic arch or carotid bodies. But even at static field strengths up to 10 T, no adverse effects on squirrel monkey EKGs have been reported. Mutagenic effects in mammals have been studied in both static magnetic fields (T_1) and gradient fields, with no adverse effects demonstrated on either adult or embryonic rodents. Extensive data have been accumulated by the National Institute for Occupational Safety and Health, the World Health Organization, and the State Department in conjunction with employees who were exposed to high levels of microwave radiation at the U.S. Embassy in Moscow, and no evidence of leukemia or other carcinogenesis has been reported. Nevertheless, in the July 22, 1982, issue of the *New England Journal of Medicine,* Milham reported increased mortality due to leukemia among men occupationally exposed to electrical and magnetic fields in Washington State from 1950 to 1979. Similar observations were reported in New York in 1987. No adverse effects from magnetic fields have been reported for personnel working with linear accelerators or high-energy physics. These individuals experience exposures of up to 2 T for short periods of time.

Gradient magnetic fields are pulsed and therefore have time-varying components that will induce electric currents in body tissues. Sufficiently intense flux densities potentially can stimulate electrically excitable cells, which would include nerve cells and muscle fibers of the heart and respiratory musculature. The most sensitive response of the body is stimulation of the retina, resulting in the sensation of flashes of light because of stimulation of the magnetic retinal phosphenes. In humans, this threshold has a minimum value of 2 to 3 T sec^{-1} at 20 to 50 Hz. Most other tissues in the body appear to be much less sensitive. Rodents have been exposed in pulse fields where the maximum rate of change has been 60 T sec^{-1}, with pulse rates as rapid as 60 msec, with no effect having been seen on heart rate, blood pressure, or respiratory rate even after 1 hr of exposure. (J. Gore and associates, *personal communication*). The typical values used in routine clinical imaging range between 0.04 T sec^{-1} and 5 T sec^{-1}, although a few subjects have experienced rates of change as high as 20 T sec^{-1}.

RF MAGNETIC FIELD

Electric currents induced in the body by exposure to RF fields are not able to excite nervous tissue. The effects of high-energy RF are confined to heating, because of resistive losses of energy in the tissues. This is a principle used in short-wave diathermy therapy. In general, chronic exposure to RF power densities producing an average power deposition of approximately 1 W kg^{-1} is considered safe, from a heat-production point of view, with a peak deposition of 8 W kg^{-1} in any gram of tissue. This power deposition is roughly equivalent to a person's basic metabolic rate, and if no heat were lost from the body, it would raise tissue temperature about 1°C in an hour. Tissues with poor blood supply, and therefore decreased rates of cooling, experience greater elevations in temperature. Those tissues with no blood supply, such as the lens of the eye, or poor blood supply, such as the testes, can be regarded as target organs for heat sensitivity. Generally, the maximum time-averaged power deposition absorbed during NMR imaging is substantially less than 1 W kg^{-1}. Therefore, this does not appear to be a problem. Metallic surgical clips or large prostheses can absorb more heat than body tissues.

How the magnetic fields-used in NMR imaging affect artificial pacemakers is not known. Many manufacturers of pacemakers include reed relays within the pacemaker to provide a means of alternating the pacemaker operation with an external magnet, which is placed on the outside of the body. Magnetic field strengths ranging from 10 to 50 G will activate the relays of these pacemakers, and thus any patients with these types of pacemakers should not be allowed to encounter field strengths greater than 3 to 5 G. In practical terms, this means that no such patients should be allowed in corridors one or two floors above or below the NMR scanner and a comparable distance on either side. Interference by weak magnetic fields can cause some modern trigger pacemakers to reverse to an asynchronous mode, and because of these concerns, people with pacemakers or large metal implants have not been imaged with NMR systems.

In conclusion, the evidence from animal experiments involving exposure to high magnetic fields and the limited studies in human patients and volunteers exposed

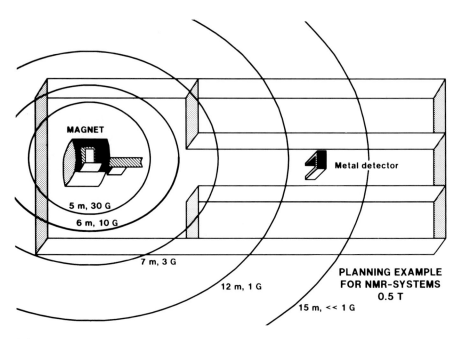

FIG. 9.2. Planning example for a 0.5-T superconducting NMR magnet. The fringe field in the long axis.

to clinical NMR imaging systems suggest that the fields used in the current systems are well below threshold for any adverse biological effect. Unless the requirements for magnetic field strength and RF power input greatly exceed the current expectations, the risk to patients undergoing MRI is likely to be substantially less than that encountered with radiographic equipment. Hazards and risks are more likely to be greater for those individuals working with the equipment or passing near it. The potential hazards that can result from the use of MRI are thus related to the following general areas: (a) injuries from ferromagnetic objects accelerated by large static magnetic fields; (b) effects on pacemakers, prostheses, and any equipment using cathode-ray tubes (CRT) that are near the magnetic field; (c) biological effects from the static magnetic field, induced currents from rapid changes in magnetic field, and heating from RF fields.

SITE-PLANNING HAZARDS

A major consideration in the decision to install an NMR imaging facility concerns the architectural requirements. The structural, mechanical, electrical, and spatial requirements of the system must be carefully evaluated to determine if the system will be placed in an existing building or a building that will be specially built for NMR imaging. The difficulty in making such determinations arises because of sev-

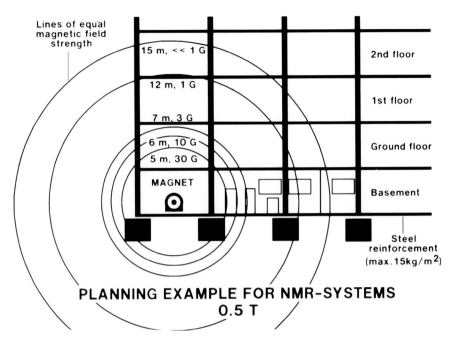

Lines of equal
magnetic field
strength

15 m, << 1 G   2nd floor

12 m, 1 G   1st floor

7 m, 3 G

6 m, 10 G   Ground floor
5 m, 30 G

MAGNET   Basement

Steel
reinforcement
(max. 15 kg/m²)

**PLANNING EXAMPLE FOR NMR-SYSTEMS
0.5 T**

FIG. 9.3. Fringe field in the transverse axis.

eral significant unknowns in NMR technology. Investigators are still evaluating the optimal field strengths for imaging applications. Without that information and answers to other questions essential to optimal system design, it is impossible to specify an ideal configuration for clinical systems that will be developed in the future. Nevertheless, certain fundamental characteristics of NMR imaging suites, specifically very strong magnetic fields and an RF transmitter-receiver, impose definite constraints on the architecture of an NMR suite. This section is designed to provide guidelines only; each institution will require special assistance to fit the NMR imager selected into the space available. Nevertheless, a general outline of the problems and questions that will be encountered should be useful.

Aside from engineering concerns, there are two general questions to be evaluated in NMR site planning:

1. What will be the effects of the magnetic field on personnel and equipment in the general environment?
2. What will be the effects of metallic structures, vehicles, and electrical equipment on the NMR system itself?

The static magnetic field of any NMR system is three-dimensional, extending above and below the magnet as well as into the surrounding space on the same level. In addition, the field is not circular, but extends farther in the direction of the magnet bore than perpendicular to the long axis. The magnetic field nevertheless

TABLE 9.1. *External influences on the magnetic field (minimum distance[a])*

1-m distance: steel reinforcement in ceiling and floor; 15 kg iron per 1 m^2
5-m distance: steel girders, highly reinforced concrete columns and beams
12-m distance: hospital transportation systems (bed transport, conveyance equipment)
12-m distance: very strong high frequency (HF) generators
15-m distance: elevators, vehicles (trucks, cars)
15-m distance: power cables, transformers

[a]Distance from the center of the magnet.

TABLE 9.2. *Influences of the magnetic field on nearby equipment (minimum distance[a])*

5-m distance: computers
6-m distance: pacemakers perpendicular to the axis of the magnet
7-m distance: television equipment, monitor screen
8.3-m distance: pacemakers along the axis of the magnet
15-m distance: X-ray unit with image-intensifier nuclear medicine (gamma camera)

[a]Distance from the center of the magnet.

falls off as the cube of the distance from the magnet system. For those planning a two-magnet suite, with an imaging magnet in combination with a spectroscopy system, the best overall approach is to align the magnets perpendicular to each other to decrease the total area of the magnetic field.

The large three-dimensional magnetic field created by the NMR magnet is the major limiting factor in system location, especially if it is to go into an existing building. Usually there are magnetic materials in the immediate environment that can distort the magnetic field of the system, degrading image quality and making NMR spectroscopy and/or electron spin resonance (ESR) spectroscopy impossible. As mentioned earlier, the magnetic field can interfere with the function of certain mechanical and electrical devices, such as CRTs and patients' pacemakers, and these magnetic-field effects must be carefully considered and minimized if possible.

In this regard, the intended ultimate purpose of the imaging system is critically important. If a basic unit capable of proton-density imaging is all that is required, then a 0.15-T resistive system will suffice, and site selection will be much simpler. However, if chemical-shift spectroscopy and perhaps hydrogen-density imaging are required, then at least a 1.5-T magnet strength will be required, greatly complicating the architectural design and requirements for controlled space.

For purposes of illustrating the kinds of concerns and problems faced in site preparation, a site model and field-strength lines are presented for a 0.5-T superconducting magnet, with field-strength lines and imaging-suite design for the same plane as the magnet (Figs. 9.2 and 9.3). Table 9.1 lists some of the influences of the external environment on the magnetic field, and Table 9.2 lists some influences of the magnetic field on the external environment. Table 9.3 lists some structural aspects of a hypothetical suite. Once again, however, these are meant only to in-

TABLE 9.3. *Structural aspects*

Weights and dimensions (0.5-T superconducting magnet)		Transport path		Maximum component weight	
NMR magnet, filled	5,300 kg	Minimum floor width	2.50	NMR magnet	4,800 kg
Dimensions (l × w × h)	2.3 × 2 × 2.54 m	Minimum floor height	2.80 m	He can	460 kg
Patient couch	300 kg	Minimum door width	2.50 m	N can	800 kg
Dimensions (l × w × h)	3.0 × 0.67 × 0.65 m	Minimum door height	2.80 m		
Recommended size of room for magnet	10 × 10 m				
Minimum size of room for magnet	5 × 8 m				
Minimum room height	3.5 m				

TABLE 9.4. Typical magnet specifications[a]

Type	0.13-T permanent magnet	0.15-T resistive magnet	0.3-T SC[b] magnet	0.5-T SC magnet	1.5–2.0-T SC magnet	Gradient-coil power supply
Size (length × height)	25' × 10' (standard shielded-room size)	6.9' × 7.5' (2.1 × 2.3 m)	7.5' × 8.2' (2.3 × 2.5 m)	7.5' × 8.2' (2.3 × 2.5 m)	7.5' × 9.8' (2.3 × 3.0 m)	2.6' × 5.9' (0.8 × 1.8 m)
Weight	1,000 tons	9,020 lb max (4,100 kg) 5,500 lb typical (2,500 kg)	8,800 lb (400 kg) 9,900 lb[c] (4,500 kg)	9,460 lb (4,300 kg) 10,560 lb (4,800 kg)	16,500 lb (7,550 kg) 17,710 lb[c] (8,050 kg)	1,100 lb (500 kg)
Minimum ceiling height	10'	9.5' (2.9 m)	9.5' (2.9 m)	9.5' (2.9 m)	14' (4.2 m)	NA
Magnetic-field distance (3 G/1 G)	None (outside shielded room)	21' (6.4 m)/ 31' (9.4 m)	27' (8.2 m)/ 37' (11.9 m)	33' (10 m)/ 47' (14.3 m)	45' (13.7 m)/ 67' (20.4 m)[e]	NA
Maximum power demand	None[d]	85 kVA max 60 kVA typical 3 phase	25 kVA max 3 phase	25 kVA max 3 phase	25 kVA max 3 phase	15–75 kVA
Cooling requirements	Room air conditioning	Water: 95 liters/min (magnet + power supply)	LN_2: 2 liters/hr LHe: 0.5 liter/hr H_2O: 3 liters/min[f]	LN_2: 2 liters/hr LHe: 0.5 liter/hr H_2O: 5 liters/min	LN_2: 2 liters/hr LNe: 0.5 liter/hr H_2O: 10 liters/min[f]	H_2O: 10 liters/min coil; 10 liters/min power supply

[a]Data from General Electric and Fonar.
[b]Superconducting.
[c]With cryogens.
[d]Electrical supply to room = 40 kW.
[e]For 1.5-T field strength.
[f]For power supply.

TABLE 9.5. *Environmental requirements: expected maximal values*

Total heat dissipation
  Permanent magnet: 0[b]
  Resistive system: 350,000 BTU/hr[c]
  Superconducting (SC) system: 100,000 BTU/hr
Altitude (max)[b]
  60,000 ft (1,826 m)
Ambient temperature range
  +60°F to +75°F (+15°C to 24°C)
  Field uniformity of permanent magnet may be very sensitive
Helium venting (SC system only)
  Normal range: 375 liters/hr
  During quench: 1.5×10^5 liters

---

[a]Data from General Electric.
[b]Not applicable to permanent magnet.
[c]Includes about 200,000 BTU/hr that is removed from magnet room by cooling water.

TABLE 9.6. *Power requirements[a]*

Permanent magnet
  Suite power requirements: 40 kW (With a permanent magnet there is no quenching nor any special power requirement. There is a minimal fringe field and limited missile effect; so site selection is relatively simple. There are no costly cryogenic expenses, and there are no moving parts except for the motorized patient bed.)
Resistive system
  Maximum power: 150 kVA
  Voltage: 480 V, 3 phase, 50–80 Hz
  Voltage tolerance: +10%, −15%
  Current (total at 480 V): momentary 175 amp; continuous 146 amp
Superconducting system
  Maximum power: 70 kVA
  Voltage: 480 V, 3 phase, 50–80 Hz
  Voltage tolerance: +10%, −15%
  Current (total at 480 V): momentary 175 amp; continuous 146 amp

---

[a]Data from General Electric, Siemens, and Fonar.

dicate the general approach to site preparation; a specific design will also depend on the specific requirements of the manufacturer of the imaging unit.

The floor plan must provide for rapid, straight-line exit from the area of the NMR magnet so that patients can be removed from the NMR suite to an area where patient monitoring and life-support equipment will operate satisfactorily in case of a medical emergency. Although not listed on the diagram, RF shielding is necessary, and for most sites at least a 90-db reduction is required. In addition, structural reinforcement is necessary for these systems, with a maximum weight of 10,000 kg.

With so many computers, terminals, image intensifiers, and other CRTs in and around most hospitals and offices, it is important to determine what the effects of magnetic fields will be on these devices. One useful approach is to measure the anisotropy, that is, unequal distortions in two dimensions of the susceptible components of the CRT (i.e., unequal distortions of the CRT image). In general, the effects are slightly greater on black-and-white CRTs than on color CRTs, but an unshielded system can expect about 2% anisotropy; however, iron shielding will decrease the effect.

Table 9.4 lists some magnet specifications for several types of NMR systems. Tables 9.5 and 9.6 list environmental and power requirements, respectively.

Chapter 10

MRI Review Quiz

Readers who now believe that they have a basic understanding of the principles of magnetic resonance should take the following quiz. If one is comfortable with the material and answers the majority of the questions correctly, the quiz can serve as a quick review of MRI and indicate those sections of the text that should be reviewed in the future.

1. The gray scale in MRI is determined predominantly by which of the following?
   1. TR and TE
   2. Electron density of the tissue
   3. The combination of bulk, structured, and bound water
   4. The echo back-scatter from structures in tissue
   A. 2 and 3 only
   B. 2 and 4 only
   C. 1 only
   D. 1 and 3 only
2. When evaluating economic value for several different MRI scanners being considered for purchase, the best type of analysis to use is:
   A. The analysis of the manufacturer, because these are highly reliable
   B. Internal rate of return
   C. Break-even analysis
   D. Net present value if a reasonable cost of capital is used
3. When a proton is precessing in a 1-T magnetic field, increasing the field by 0.001 T causes the precessional frequency to:
   A. decrease
   B. stay the same because the field change is small
   C. increase
   D. any of the above, depending on conditions
4. The magnetic field strength of the earth versus the magnetic field strength of a typical magnetic resonance scanner is:
   A. 0.5/2,000 Larmor
   B. 0.5/15,000 G
   C. 2/1,000 Fourier
   D. 2/100 G
5. T_1 and T_2 are two decay constants associated with NMR:
   A. T_1 is equal to $2T_2$
   B. T_1 is less than or equal to T_2

C. T_1 is greater than or equal to T_2
D. $2T_1$ equals T_2
6. The Larmor (resonant) frequency, ω_0, is determined by:
   A. the magnetic field strength
   B. the nuclear-decay constant
   C. the magnetogyric ratio
   D. the magnetogyric ratio and magnetic field strength
7. For hydrogen (protons, ^{1}H) placed in a 0.1-T (1,000-G) field, the resonant frequency will be:
   A. 0.98 MHz
   B. 4.26 MHz
   C. 6.39 MHz
   D. 0.65 MHz
8. What is resonating in MRI?
   A. the sample atoms
   B. the sample molecules
   C. biopolymers larger than 40,000 molecular weight
   D. only water and fat in the patient
9. The purpose of the gradient-magnetic-field coils is to:
   A. direct the flow of protons
   B. excite the emission of radio-wave photons
   C. provide spatial localization of NMR signals
   D. cause emission of radio-wave photons
10. In comparison with other techniques such as CT and radiography, the most important characteristic of MRI is:
   A. improved cost
   B. improved contrast resolution
   C. improved spatial resolution
   D. improved speed
11. Magnetic resonance is a phenomenon that occurs when a static external magnetic field is applied to a tissue, and it occurs in all atoms with:
   A. protons
   B. electrons
   C. neutrons
   D. unpaired protons, electrons, or neutrons

Answers to MRI quiz:

1. D	5. C	9. C
2. D	6. D	10. B
3. C	7. B	11. D
4. B	8. A	

MRI Glossary

Absorption line. A relative peak in the frequency spectrum from NMR spectroscopy that corresponds to a characteristic absorption of the radio-frequency (RF) pulse.

Adiabatic fast passage. A technique used to invert net tissue magnetization by sweeping the magnetic field (or RF spectrum) through the resonant frequency.

American College of Radiology imaging terms. See Pulse sequence, Interpulse time, Repetition time (TR), Inversion time (T_1), and Echo time (TE).

Angular frequency (ω). Rotational frequency, usually expressed in hertz (Hz). Nuclear particles spin around a central axis. The measure of this rotational motion is called *angular momentum*. Other atomic particles, especially electrons, may also possess orbital angular momentum as well as spin angular momentum.

Chemical shift. In NMR spectroscopy, chemical shifts are observable as slightly displaced resonant peaks in higher-resolution (field homogeneity $1/10^6$) NMR systems and result from the differential shielding effect of electrons orbiting in the molecule. (These chemical shifts, in other words, are due to the regional magnetic forces within the molecular environment.)

Coherence. Term used in NMR to describe the magnetic moments of nuclear particles that are rotating or precessing in phase.

Diamagnetic. Pertains to a sample in which the internal induced magnetic field is in the opposite direction to and usually much weaker than the external magnetic field.

Echo time (TE). Time between the middle of a 90° pulse and the middle of spin-echo production. For multiple echoes, use TE_1, TE_2, etc.

Fast Fourier transformation (FFT). A fast and efficient algorithm for calculating Fourier-transform analyses on a digital computer.

Fourier transformation (FT). A mathematical algorithm that is capable of converting a complex waveform into either a signal that is observable as amplitude versus time or a signal of amplitude versus frequency. The process is a representation of the complex wave function by a sum of sine and cosine. The FFT is a somewhat shortened version of the longer FT.

Gauss (G). A unit of magnetic field strength or magnetic flux density. In MRI, magnetic field strengths usually are expressed as kilogauss (10^3 G).

Gradient magnetic field. A magnetic field whose strength varies along a linear direction.

Gyromagnetic ratio (γ). A parameter relating the nuclear magnetic frequency to the static magnetic field strength, characteristic or specific for each particular nuclear species. It is also called the *magnetogyric* and is defined by the Larmor equation.

Hertz (Hz). The unit of frequency measurement indicating the number of complete cycles completed in 1 sec.

Image acquisition time. To calculate acquisition time: total acquisition time = (TR) × (acquisition matrix) × (2) × (number of signal averages) × number of slices.

Interpulse times. Times between successive RF pulses used in pulse sequences. Particularly important are the inversion time (TI) in inversion-recovery and the time between a 90° pulse and subsequent 180° pulse to produce a spin-echo. This interval will be approximately one-half the spin-echo time (TE). The time between repetitions of pulse sequences is the repetition time (TR).

Inversion-recovery. An imaging sequence involving a 180°-to-90° RF pulse sequence that provides T_1 discrimination.

Inversion time (TI). The time between the middle of an inverting RF pulse and the middle of a subsequent 90° pulse to detect the amount of longitudinal magnetization.

Larmor relation. Larmor frequency is the resonant frequency in a given magnetic field, where the relationship for hydrogen is 42.58 MHz/T.

Lorentzian line. A radio-frequency absorption line obtained from a spectroscopic experiment with a narrow peak and long tail.

Magnetic dipole. Essentially a bar magnet, or any north and south magnetic poles that are separated by some distance. Spinning charged particles can create magnetic-dipole moments.

Magnetic moment. The torque or force exerted in a magnetic field of given strength when the axis of the magnet is at right angles to the field. Nuclear magnetic moment is the magnetic moment associated with spinning charged nuclear particles.

Magnetization. In NMR imaging, magnetization generally refers to net tissue magnetization, which is the net effort of the ensemble of large numbers of protons, a slight majority of which are oriented parallel to the static magnetic field. It is this slight excess of parallel protons that confers net tissue magnetization to the tissue or sample being imaged.

Nuclear magnetic resonance (NMR). The resonant emission and absorption of radio-frequency electromagnetic energy by nuclei in a static external magnetic field. The resonant frequency of absorption is directly proportional to the strength of the external field.

Paramagnetic. Pertains to a sample in which the internal induced magnetic field is the same direction as the applied external field. This property, however, is not retained when the external field is removed.

Paramagnetic atoms. Atoms that slightly increase a magnetic field when they are placed within it are referred to as paramagnetic. In general, such an atom has an odd number of electrons, with a partially filled inner electron shell.

Precession (wobbling). A spinning top in the earth's gravitational field or a proton in an external magnetic field wobbles or precesses around its axis. The frequency of precession ω in NMR imaging is given by the Larmor equation $\omega = \gamma B$, where γ is the gyromagnetic ratio and B is the static magnetic field.

Probe. In an NMR spectroscopy system, the part that contains the sample and the RF coils is referred to as the probe.

Pulse sequences. Sets of RF (and/or gradient) magnetic-field pulses and time spacings between these pulses; used in conjunction with gradient magnetic fields and NMR signal reception to produce NMR images.

Quenching. Loss (usually unexpected) of the near-absolute-zero temperature induced by the surrounding liquid helium in a superconducting magnet. When superconductivity is lost, the magnet will acutely become resistive.

Radio frequency (RF). The portion of the electromagnetic spectrum containing the radio waves with wavelengths between 10 and 10^4 m and frequency 10^4 to 10^9 Hz.

Radio-frequency (RF) coil. The antenna used for transmitting or irradiating RF pulses and receiving the emitted signal in NMR imaging systems.

Radio-frequency (RF) pulse. The pulse, usually of short duration, generated by an RF oscillator and transmitted by an RF coil.

Relaxation. The process by which molecules move between high energy states and low energy states. The method of relaxation depends on the physical state of the tissue being studied. In NMR, it is the time required for magnetization to return to equilibrium after an RF pulse.

Repetition time (TR). The period of time between the beginning of a pulse sequence and the beginning of a succeeding (essentially identical) pulse sequence.

Resonance. The exchange of energy at specified frequencies. In NMR, it is the process by which nuclei absorb radio-frequency energy that causes the protons to flip between upper and lower or parallel and antiparallel energy states.

Rotating frame. A concept originally applied by Tesla in which a frame of reference rotates with the precessing nuclear moments. In this system, the motion of the precessing magnetization is in some respects easier to describe.

Shim coils. Flat wire coils used to produce small magnetic gradients in an NMR system to correct field inhomogeneities. These are used extensively in fitting magnets into structures that were not designed for NMR systems.

Signal-to-noise ratio. In NMR imaging, background noise increases in the coil as the square root of the frequency; however, the nuclear signal increases as the frequency squared (f^2). The ideal signal-to-noise ratio is proportional to $f^{3/2}$. Theoretically, at higher field strengths, this relationship once was thought to change because of the increased radio-frequency adsorption that was due to the electrical conductivity of the body. Recently, however, experiments have shown that proton imaging can be performed at 1.5 T, and many of these theoretical concerns may not have practical consequences.

Spectrum. The spectrum in NMR is the display of the relative radio-frequency adsorption peaks in the frequency domain plotted as functions of their resonant frequencies.

Spin. A property of a spinning particle, electron, neutron, or proton, that determines its magnetic moment. The spin of an electron or proton is one-half.

Spin-echo. An NMR signal that occurs at fixed intervals after a perturbation and results from phase coherence. The signal has a crescendo–descrescendo character and is called the *echo* or *spin-echo* signal.

T_1 relaxation time. Also called *spin-lattice* or *longitudinal relaxation time.* This is the exponential time constant at which the component of magnetization parallel to the external field returns to equilibrium conditions. This decay results from the interaction of a nucleus (spin) with its physical surroundings (lattice) and is therefore called spin-lattice relaxation.

T_2 relaxation time. Also called *spin-spin* or *transverse relaxation time.* This is the exponential time constant that the component of magnetization that is perpendicular to the external field requires to return to equilibrium conditions in a homogeneous magnetic field. It results from the decay of coherence in the perpendicular plane and is the result of interactions of the spinning nuclei with the spin of identical nuclei pointing in the opposite direction and hence is called spin-spin relaxation.

T_2^*. Effective transverse relaxation time in a nonhomogeneous field ($T_2^* < T_2$).

Tesla. The usual unit of magnetic field strength, equal to 10,000 G.

Three-dimensional and two-dimensional Fourier transformation (2DFT and 3DFT). An imaging technique in which spatial information is phase-encoded in the precessing nuclei by selective use of gradient magnetic fields.

Zeugmatography. A term originally used by Lauterbur, taken from the Greek root *zeugma,* meaning "to join together." This word was chosen to indicate the use of electromagnetic waves and NMR as the yoke between the two forms of energy in this type of imaging.

Bibliography

CHAPTERS 1 to 4

1. Abragam, A. (1961): *Principles of Nuclear Magnetism.* Clarendon Press, Oxford.
2. Andrew, E. R. (1969): *Nuclear Magnetic Resonance.* Cambridge University Press, Cambridge, U.K.
3. Becker, E. D. (1980): *High Resolution NMR—Theory and Chemical Applications,* ed. 2. Academic Press, New York.
4. Bloch, F. (1946): Nuclear induction. *Phys. Rev.,* 70 (7,8).
5. Bradley, W. G. (1982): NMR tomography. Diasonics interactive education program.
6. Budinger, T. F., and Margulis, A. R. (1986): *Magnetic Resonance Imaging and Spectroscopy, A Primer.* SMRM, Berkeley.
7. Carr, H. Y., and Purcell, E. M. (1954): Effects of diffusion on free precession in nuclear resonance experiments. *Phys. Rev.,* 94 (3).
8. Carrington, A., and McLachlan, A. D. (1967): *Introduction to Magnetic Resonance.* Harper & Row, New York.
9. Damadian, R. (1971): Tumor detection by nuclear magnetic resonance. *Science,* 171:1151–1153.
10. Damadian, R., Goldsmith, M., and Minhoff, L. (1977): NMR in cancer: XVI Fonar image of the live human body. *Physiol. Chem. Phys.,* 9.
11. Fullerton, G.D. (1982): Basic concepts for nuclear magnetic resonance imaging. *Magn. Reson. Imag.,* 1:39–55.
12. Gadian, D. G. (1982): *Nuclear Magnetic Resonance and Its Applications to Living Systems.* Oxford University Press, Oxford.
13. Kneeland, J. B., Jesmanowicz, A., Froncisz, W., Grist, T. M., and Hyde, J. (1986): High-resolution MR imaging using loop-gap resonators. *Radiology* 158:247–250.
14. Lauterbur, P. C. (1973): Image formation by induced local interactions: examples employing nuclear magnetic resonance. *Nature,* 242(5394):190.
15. Mansfield, P. (1981): Critical evaluation of NMR imaging techniques. *Proc. ISNMRI,* 81–87.
16. Mansfield, P. (1977): Multi-planar image formation using NMR spin echoes. *J. Phys. C: Solid State Phys.,* 10.
17. Mansfield, P., and Morris, P. G. (1982): *NMR Imaging in Biomedicine,* pp. 155–201. Academic Press, New York.
18. Oldendorf, W. H. (1982): NMR imaging: Its potential clinical impact. *Hosp. Pract.,* 114–124.
19. Oldendorf, W. H. (1980): *The Quest for an Image of Brain.* Raven Press, New York.
20. Partain, C. L., James, A. E., Rollo, F. D., and Price, R. R. (1983): *Nuclear Magnetic Resonance (NMR) Imaging.* W. B. Saunders, Philadelphia.
21. Purcell, E. M., Taurry, H. C., and Pound, R. V. (1946): Resonance absorption by nuclear magnetic moments in a solid. *Phys. Rev.,* 69:37.
22. Pykett, I. L. (1982): NMR imaging in medicine. *Sci. Am.,* 246:78–88.
23. Pykett, I. L., Newhouse, J. H., Buonanno, F. S., Brady, T. J., Goldman, M. R., Kistler, J. P., and Pohost, G. M. (1982): Principles of nuclear magnetic resonance imaging. *Radiology,* 143:157–168.
24. Roschmann, P., Tischler, R. (1986): Surface coil proton MR imaging at 2 T. *Radiology,* 161:251–255.
25. Ross, B. D., Radda, G. K., Gadian, D. G., Rocker, G., Esiri, M., and Falconer-Smith, J. (1981): Examination of a case of suspected McArdle's syndrome by ^{31}P nuclear magnetic resonance. *N. Engl. J. Med.,* 304:1338–1342.
26. Schenck, J. F., Hart, H. R., Jr., Foster, T. H., Edelstein, W. A., Hussain, M.A. (1986): High resolution magnetic resonance imaging using surface coils. In: *Magnetic Resonance Annual 1986,* edited by H. Y. Kressel. Raven Press, New York.

27. Singer, J. R. (1978): Nuclear magnetic resonance diffusion and flow measurements and an introduction to spin phase graphing. *J. Phys. E: Sci. Instrum.*, 2:18–21.
28. Steiner, R. E. (1986): Present and future clinical position of magnetic resonance imaging. *Magn. Reson. Med.*, 3:473–490.
29. Sutherland, R. J., Hutchinson, J. M. S. (1973): Magnetic resonance zeugmatography. *Nature (Lond.)*, 242:190.

CHAPTER 5

1. Bottomley, P. A., Foster, T. H., Argersinger, R. E., et al. (1984): A review of normal tissue hydrogen NMR relaxation times and relaxation mechanisms from 1–100 MHz: Dependence on tissue type, NMR frequency, temperature, species, excision, and age. *Med. Phys.*, 11:425–448.
2. Brant-Zawadzki, M., Bartkowski, H. M., Ortendahl, D. A., et al. (1984): NMR in experimental cerebral edema: Value of T_1 and T_2 calculations. *AJNR*, 5:125–129.
3. Brown, J. J., and van Sonnenberg, E. (1986): MR characterization of biologic tissues and fluids. *Applied Radiology*, May/June:73–76.
4. Brown, J. J., van Sonnenberg, E., Gerber, K. H., et al. (1985): Magnetic resonance relaxation times of percutaneously obtained normal and abnormal body fluids. *Radiology*, 154:727–731.
5. Brown, M. S., and Gore, J. C. (1987): NMR relaxation in hydrogels: A model for tissues. In: *Abstracts of the SMRI*, 5(Suppl. 1):88.
6. Engelstad, B. L., and Wolf, G. (1987): Most promising MR contrast agents affect signal by enhancing relaxation. *Diagnostic Imaging*, March:145–156.
7. Engelstad, B. L., and Wolf, G. (1987): Principles of magnetic resonance contrast agents. *Magn. Reson. Imag.*, (*in press*).
8. Engelstad, B. D., White, D. I., and Moseley, M. E. (1987):Pharmacologic selection of focal phosphorus-31 signal using iron-containing superparamagnetic particulates. Presented at SMRI meeting, San Antonio, March.
9. Foster, M. A., Rimmington, J. E., and Mallard, J. R. (1987): Variation in tissue T_1 relaxation time with measurement of temperature and frequency. An in vitro study of rat tissues. In: *Abstracts of the SMRI*, 5(Suppl. 1):90.
10. Fullerton, G. D. (1987): Physiologic basis of contrast in MRI. *Magn. Reson. Imag. (in press)*.
11. Fung, B. M. (1977): Correlation of relaxation times with water content in muscle and brain tissues. *Biochim. Biophys. Acta*, 497:317–322.
12. Kilgore, D. P., Breger, R. K., Daniels, D. L., Pojunas, K. W., Williams, A. L., and Haughton, V. M. (1986): Cranial tissues: Normal MR appearance after intravenous injection of Gd-DTPA. *Radiology*, 160:757–761.
13. Lauterbur, P. C., Mendoca-Dias, M. H., and Rudin, A. M. (1978): Augmentation of tissue water proton spin lattice relaxation rates by in vivo addition of paramagnetic ions. In: *Frontiers of Biological Energetics*. Academic Press, New York.
14. Runge, V. M., Claussen, C. Relix, R., and James, A. E. (editors) (1986): *Contrast Agents in Magnetic Resonance Imaging*. Excerpta Medica, Princeton, N.J.
15. White, D. W., Engelstad, B. L., Brasch, R. C., and Weiner, M. W. (1986): Relaxation agents for in vivo ^{31}P NMR: Effects of some Gd(III) chelates on the ^{31}P NMR spectra and relaxation times of ATP, creatine phosphate and inorganic phosphate in vitro. Presented at SMRM meeting, Montreal (abstr.).
16. Wolf, G. L., Sullenberger, P. C., and Bickerstaff, K. J. (1987): The effects of temperature upon proton relaxation rates in biological tissues. In: *Abstract of the SMRI*, 5(Suppl. 1):91.

CHAPTER 6

MRI of the Head and Neck

1. Atlas, S. W., Grossman, R. I., Goldberg, H. I., et al. (1986): MR diagnosis of acute disseminated encephalomyelitis. *JCAT*, 10(5):798–801.

2. Atlas, S. W., Zimmerman, R. A., Bilaniuk, L. T., et al. (1986): Corpus collosum and limbic system: Neuroanatomic MR evaluation of developmental anomalies. *Radiology,* 160:355–362.
3. Berger, P. E., Atkinson, D., Wilson, W. J., and Wiltse, L. (1986): High resolution surface coil magnetic resonance imaging of the spine: Normal and pathologic anatomy. *RadioGraphics,* 6(4):573–602.
4. Darwin, R. H., Drayer, B. P., Riederer, S. J., et al. (1986): T_2 estimates in healthy and diseased brain tissue: A comparison using various MR pulse sequences. *Radiology,* 160:375–381.
5. Edwards, M. K., Farlow, M. R., and Stevens, J. C. (1986): Multiple sclerosis: MRI and clinical correlation. *AJR,* 147:571–574.
6. Franken, E. A., Jr., Berbaum, K. S., Dunn, V., Smith, W. L., et al. (1986): Impact of MR imaging on clinical diagnosis and management: A prospective study. *Radiology,* 161:377–380.
7. Kirkpatrick, J. B., and Hayman, L. A. (1987): White-matter lesions in MR imaging of clinically healthy brains of elderly subjects: Possible pathologic basis. *Radiology,* 162:509–511.
8. Kucharczyk, W., Davis, D. O., Kelly, W. M., et al. (1986): Pituitary adenomas: High-resolution MR imaging at 1.5 T. *Radiology,* 161:761–765.
9. Kucharczyk, W., Kelly, W. M., Davis, D. O., et al. (1986): Intracranial lesions: flow-related enhancement on MR images using time-of-flight effects. *Radiology,* 161:767–772.
10. Le Bihan, D., Breton, E., Lallemand, D., et al. (1986): MR imaging of intravoxel incoherent motions: Application to diffusion and perfusion in neurologic disorders. *Radiology,* 161:401–407.
11. Luyten, P. R., den Hollander, J. A., et al. (1986): Observation of metabolites in the human brain by MR spectroscopy. *Radiology,* 161:795–798.
12. McArdle, C. B., Richardson, C. J., Nicholas, D. A., et al. (1987): Developmental features of the neonatal brain: MR imaging, part 1 and 2. *Radiology,* 162:223–229.
13. Mintz, M. C., Grossman, R. I., Isaacson, G., et al. (1987): MR imaging of fetal brain. *JCAT,* 11(1):120–123.
14. New, P. F. J., Ojemann, R. G., Davis, K. R., et al. (1986): MR and CT of occult vascular malformations of the brain. *AJR,* 147:985–993.
15. Nose, T., Enomoto, T., Hyodo, A., et al. (1987): Case report: Intracerebral hematoma developing during MR examination. *JCAT,* 11(1):184–187.
16. Nowell, M. A., Hackney, D. B., Zimmerman, R. A., et al. (1987): Immature brain: Spin-echo pulse sequence parameters for high-contrast MR imaging. *Radiology,* 162:272–273.
17. Olsen, W. L., Dillon, W. P., Kelly, W. M., et al. (1987): MR imaging of paragangliomas. *AJR,* 148:201–204.
18. Rubin, J. B., and Enzmann, D. R. (1987): Imaging of spinal CSF pulsation by 2DFT magnetic resonance: Significance during clinical imaging. *AJNR,* 8:297–306.
19. Rubin, J. B., and Enzmann, D. R. (1987): Harmonic modulation of proton MR precessional phase by pulsatile motion: Origin of spinal CSF flow phenomenon. *AJNR,* 8:307–318.
20. Rubin, J. B., Enzmann, D. R., and Wright, A. (1987): CSF gated spine MRI: Theory and clinical implementation. *Radiology, (in press).*
21. Sherman, J. L., Citrin, C. M., Gangarosa, R. E., and Bowen, B. J. (1987): The MR appearance of CSF flow in patients with ventriculomegaly. *AJR,* 148:193–199.
22. Spagnoli, M. V., Goldberg, H. I., Grossman, R. I., et al. (1986): Intracranial meningiomas: High-field MR imaging. *Radiology,* 161:369–375.
23. Wilson, D. A., and Steiner, R. E. (1986): Periventribular leukomalacia: Evaluation with MR imaging. *Radiology,* 160:507–511.
24. Young, I. R., Khenia, S., Thomas, D. G. T., Davis, C. H., et al. (1987): Clinical magnetic susceptibility mapping of the brain. *JCAT,* 11(1):2–6.
25. Zimmerman, R. A., Bilaniuk, L. T., Hackney, D. B., et al. (1987): Paranasal sinus hemorrhage: Evaluation with MR imaging. *Radiology,* 162:499–503.

Thorax

1. Axel, L., Kressel, H. Y., Thickman, D., et al. (1983): NMR imaging of the chest at 0.12 T: Initial clinical experience with a resistive magnet. *AJR,* 141:1157–1162.
2. Didier, D., and Higgins, C. B. (1986): Estimation of pulmonary vascular resistance by MRI in patients with congenital cardiovascular shunt lesions. *AJR,* 146:919–924.

3. Dinsmore, R. E., Wedeen, V. J., Miller, S. W., et al. (1986): MRI of dissection of the aorta: Recognition of the intimal tear and differential flow velocities. *AJR*, 146:1286–1288.
4. Edelman, R. R., Thompson, R., Kantor, H., et al. (1987): Cardiac function: Evaluation with fast-echo MR imaging. *Radiology*, 162:611–615.
5. Fisher, M. R., and Higgins, C. B. (1986): Central thrombi in pulmonary arterial hypertension detected by MR imaging. *Radiology*, 158:223–226.
6. Fletcher, B. D., and Jacobstein, M. D. (1986): MRI of congenital abnormalities of the great arteries. *AJR*, 146:941–948.
7. Glazer, H. S., Lee, J. K. T., Levitt, R. G., et al. (1985): Radiation fibrosis: Differentiation from recurrent tumor by MR imaging. *Radiology*, 156:721–726.
8. Higgins, C. B. (1986): Overview of MR of the heart—1986. *AJR*, 146:907–918.
9. Huber, D. J., Kirkman, R. L., Kupiec-Weglinski, J., et al. (1985): The detection of cardiac allograft rejection by alterations in proton NMR relaxation times. *Invest. Radiol.* 20:796–802.
10. Moore, E. H., Webb, W. R., Muller, N., and Sollitto, R. (1986): MRI of pulmonary airspace disease: Experimental model and preliminary clinical results. *AJR*, 146:1123–1128.
11. O'Connell, D. M., and Yousef, S. J. (1984): Breast MRI shows promise in diagnosis of lesions. *Diagnostic Imaging*, 136–138.
12. O'Donovan, P. B., Ross, J. S., Sivak, E. D., et al. (1984): Magnetic resonance imaging of the thorax: The advantages of coronal and sagittal planes. *AJR*, 143:1183–1188.
13. Rholl, K. S., Levitt, R. G., Glazer, H. S., et al. (1986): Oblique magnetic resonance imaging of the cardiovascular system. *RadioGraphics*, 6(2):177–188.
14. Ross, J. S., O'Donovan, P. B., Novoa, R., et al. (1984): Magnetic resonance of the chest: initial experience with imaging and in vivo T_1 and T_2 calculations. *Radiology*, 152:95–101.
15. Skalina, S., Kundel, H. L., Wolf, G., and Marshall, B. (1984): The effect of pulmonary edema on proton nuclear magnetic resonance relaxation times. *Invest. Radiol.*, 19:7–9.
16. Stein, M. G., Crues, J. V., III, Bradley, W. G., Jr., et al. (1986): MR imaging of pulmonary emboli: An experimental study in dogs. *AJR*, 147:1133–1137.
17. Tascholakoff, D., Higgins, C. B., Sechtem, U., et al. (1986): MRI of reperfused myocardial infarct in dogs. *AJR*, 146:925–930.
18. Valk, P. E., Hale, J. D., Crooks, L. E., et al. (1986): MR imaging of aortoiliac atherosclerosis with 3D image reconstruction. *JCAT*, 10(3):439–444.
19. Valk, P. E., Hale, J. D., Kaufman, L., et al. (1985): MR imaging of the aorta with three-dimensional vessel reconstruction: Validation by angiography. *Radiology*, 157:721–725.
20. Webb, W. R., Gamsu, G., Stark, D. D., and Moore, E. H. (1984): Magnetic resonance imaging of the normal and abnormal pulmonary hila. *Radiology*, 152:89–94.
21. Webb, W. R., Jensen, B. G., Gamsu, G., et al. (1984): Coronal magnetic resonance imaging of the chest: Normal and abnormal. *Radiology*, 153:729–735.
22. Wexler, H. R., Nicholson, R. L., Prato, F. S., et al. (1985): Quantitation of lung water by nuclear magnetic resonance imaging. A preliminary study. *Invest. Radiol.*, 20:583–590.

MRI of Blood and Cardiovascular Structures

1. Axel, L. (1984): Blood flow effects in magnetic resonance imaging. *AJR*, 143:1157–1166.
2. Bradley, W. G., Jr., and Waluch, V. (1985): Blood flow: Magnetic resonance imaging. *Radiology*, 154:443–450.
3. Bradley, W. G., Jr., Waluch, V., Lai, K., et al. (1984): The appearance of rapidly flowing blood on magnetic resonance images. *AJR*, 143:1167–1174.
4. Buckwalter, K. A., Aisen, A. M., Dilworth, L. R., et al. (1986): Gated cardiac MRI: Ejection-fraction determination using the right anterior oblique view. *AJR*, 147:33–37.
5. Burbank, F., Parish, D., and Wexler, L. (1987): Echocardiographic-like angled views of the heart by magnetic resonance imaging. (*in press*).
6. Didier, D., Higgins, C. B., Fisher, M. R., et al. (1986): Congenital heart disease: Gated MR imaging in 72 patients. *Radiology*, 158:227–235.
7. Diethelm, L., Dery, R., Lipton, M. J., and Higgins, C. B. (1987): Atrial-level shunts: Sensitivity and specificity of MR in diagnosis. *Radiology*, 162:181–186.
8. Dinsmore, R. E., Wismer, G. L., Miller, S. W., et al. (1985): Magnetic resonance imaging of the heart using image planes oriented to cardiac axes: Experience with 100 cases. *AJR*, 145:1177–1183.

9. Feinberg, D. A., Crooks, L., Hoenninger, J., III, et al. (1984): Pulsatile blood velocity in human arteries displayed by magnetic resonance imaging. *Radiology,* 153:177–180.
10. Feinberg, D. A., Crooks, L. E., Sheldon, P., et al. (1985): Magnetic resonance imaging the velocity vector components of fluid flow. *Magn. Reson. Med.,* 2:555–566.
11. Kaul, S., Wismer, G. L., Brady, T. J., et al. (1986): Measurement of normal left heart dimensions using optimally oriented MR images. *AJR,* 146:75–79.
12. Kucharczyk, W., Brant-Zawadzki, M., Lemme-Plaghos, L., et al. (1985): MR technology: Effect of even-echo rephasing on calculated T_2 values and T_2 images. *Radiology,* 157:95–101.
13. Mills, C. M., Brant-Zawadzki, M., Crooks, L. E., et al. (1984): Nuclear magnetic resonance: Principles of blood flow imaging. *AJR,* 142:165–170.
14. Mills, T. C., Ortendahl, D. A., Hylton, N. M., et al. (1987): Partial flip angle MR imaging. *Radiology,* 162:531–539.
15. Nishimura, D. G., Macovski, A., Pauly, J. M., and Conolly, S. M. (1987): MR angiography by selective inversion recovery. *Magn. Reson. Med.,* 4:193–202.
16. Perman, W. H., Moran, P. R., Moran, R. A., and Bernstein, M. A. (1986): Artifacts from pulsatile flow in MR imaging. *JCAT,* 10(3):473–483.
17. Rokey, R., Verani, M. S., Bolli, R., et al. (1986): Myocardial infarct size quantification by MR imaging early after coronary artery occlusion in dogs. *Radiology,* 158:771–774.
18. Sechtem, U., Pflugfelder, P. W., White, R. D., et al. (1987): Cine MR imaging: Potential for the evaluation of cardiovascular function. *AJR,* 148:239–246.
19. Sechtem, U., Tscholakoff, D., and Higgins, C. B. (1986): MRI of the abnormal pericardium. *AJR,* 147:245–252.
20. Stahlberg, F., Nordell, B., Ericsson, A., et al. (1986): Quantitative study of flow dependence in NMR images at low flow velocities. *JCAT,* 10(6):1006–1015.
21. von Schulthess, G. K., and Higgins, C. B. (1985): Blood flow imaging with MR: Spin-phase phenomena. *Radiology,* 157:687–695.
22. Waluch, V., and Bradley, W. G. (1984): NMR even echo rephasing in slow laminar flow. *JCAT,* 8(4):594–598.
23. Wedeen, V. J., and Chao, Y. S. (1987): Rapid three-dimensional angiography with undersampled MR imaging. *JCAT,* 11(1):24–30.
24. Wehrli, F. W., Shimakawa, A., Gullberg, G. T., and MacFall, J. R. (1986): Time-of-flight MR flow imaging: Selective saturation recovery with gradient refocusing. *Radiology,* 160:781–785.
25. Wehrli, F. W., Shimakawa, A., MacFall, J. R., et al. (1985): MR imaging of venous and arterial flow by a selective saturation-recovery spin echo (SSRSE) method. *JCAT,* 9(3):537–545.
26. White, E. M., Edelman, R. R., Wedeen, V. J., and Brady, T. J. (1986): Intravascular signal in MR imaging: Use of phase display for differentiation of blood-flow signal from intraluminal disease. *Radiology,* 161:245–249.
27. Winkler, M. L., and Higgins, C. B. (1986): MRI of perivalvular infectious pseudoaneurysms. *AJR,* 147:253–256.

Blood Hemorrhage and Iron

1. Cohen, M. D., McGuire, W., Cory, D. A., and Smith, J. A. (1986): MR appearance of blood and blood products: An in vitro study. *AJR,* 146:1293–1297.
2. Drayer, B., Burger, P., Darwin, R., et al. (1986): MRI of brain iron. *AJR,* 147:103–110.
3. Erdman, W. A., Weinreb, J. C., Cohen, J. M., et al. (1986): Venous thrombosis: Clinical and experimental MR imaging. *Radiology,* 161:233–238.
4. Goldberg, H. I., Grossman, R. I., Gomori, J. M., et al. (1986): Cervical internal carotid artery dissecting hemorrhage: Diagnosis using MR. *Radiology,* 158:157–161.
5. Gomori, J. M., Grossman, R. I., Goldberg, H. I., et al. (1985): Intracranial hematomas: Imaging by high-field MR. *Radiology,* 157:87–93.
6. Hackney, D. B., Lesnick, J. E., Zimmerman, R. A., et al. (1986): MR identification of bleeding site in subarachnoid hemorrhage with multiple intracranial aneurysms. *JCAT,* 10(5):878–880.
7. Macchi, P. J., Grossman, R. I., Gomori, J. M., et al. (1986): High field MR imaging of cerebral venous thrombosis. *JCAT,* 10(1):10–15.
8. Rapoport, S., Sostman, H. D., Pope, C., et al. (1987): Venous clots: Evaluation with MR imaging. *Radiology,* 162:527–530.

9. Rubin, J. I., Gomori, J. M., Grossman, R. I., et al. (1987): High-field MR imaging of extra-cranial hematomas. *AJR*, 148:813–817.

Abdomen and Pelvis

1. Baker, L. L., Hajek, P. C., Burkhard, T. K., et al. (1987): MR imaging of the scrotum: Normal anatomy. *Radiology*, 163:89–92.
2. Falke, T. H. M., te Strake, L., Sandler, M. P., et al. (1987): Magnetic resonance imaging of the adrenal glands. *RadioGraphics* 7(2):343–370.
3. Hricak, H. (1986): MRI of the female pelvis: A review. *AJR*, 146:1115–1122.
4. Ogle, P. L. (1986): Fast scanning helps make abdominal MRI of more than academic interest. *Diagnostic Imaging*, 137–146.
5. Seidenwurm, D., Smathers, R. L., Lo, R., et al. (1987): Magnetic resonance imaging of the testes and scrotum at 1.5 Tesla. *Radiology*, 164:393–398.
6. Sommer, F. G., McNeal, J. E., and Carrol, C. L. (1986): MR depiction of zonal anatomy of the prostate at 1.5 T. *JCAT*, 10(6):983–989.
7. Weekes, R. G., Berquist, T. H., McLeod, R. A., and Zimmer, W. D. (1985): Magnetic resonance imaging of soft-tissue tumors: Comparison with computed tomography. *Mag. Reson. Imag.*, 3(4):345–352.
8. Worthington, J. L., Balfe, D. M., Lee, J. K. T., et al. (1986): Uterine neoplasms: MR imaging. *Radiology*, 159:725–730.
9. Yuasa, Y., and Kundel, H. L. (1985): Magnetic resonance imaging following unilateral occlusion of the renal circulation in rabbits. *Radiology*, 154:151:156.

Extremities and Joints

1. Aisen, A. M., Martel, W., Braunstein, E. M., et al. (1986): MRI and CT evaluation of primary bone and soft-tissue tumors. *AJR*, 146:749–756.
2. Beltran, J., et al. (1986): Joint effusions, MR imaging. *Radiology*, 158:133–137.
3. Beltran, J., et al. (1986): The knee: Surface-coil MR imaging at 1.5 T. *Radiology*, 159:747–751.
4. Christiansen, E. L., Thompson, J. R., Hasso, A. N., and Hinshaw, D. B., Jr. (1986): Correlative thin section temporomandibular joint anatomy and computed tomography. *RadioGraphics*, 6(4):703–723.
5. Drace, J. E., Young, S. W., and Enzmann, D. R. (1987): The MRI ultrastructure of the TMJ meniscus: Diagnostic landmarks and pitfalls of interpretation. (*in press*).
6. Harms, S. E., Wilk, R. M., Wolford, L. M., et al. (1985): The temporomandibular joint: Magnetic resonance imaging using surface coils. *Radiology*, 157:133–136.
7. Hudson, T. M., Hamlin, D. J., Enneking, W. F., et al. (1985): Magnetic resonance imaging of bone and soft tissue tumors: Early experience in 31 patients compared with computed tomography. *Skeletal Radiology*, 13:134–146.
8. Kangarloo, H., Dietrich, R. B., Taira, R. T., et al. (1986): MR imaging of bone marrow in children. *JCAT*, 10(2): 205–209.
9. Koenig, H., Lenz, M., and Sauter, R. (1986): Temporal bone region: High-resolution MR imaging using surface coils. *Radiology*, 159:191–194.
10. Kulkarni, M. V., Drolshagen, L. F., Kaye, J. J., et al. (1986): MR imaging of hemophiliac arthropathy. *JCAT*, 10(3):445–449.
11. Mitchell, D. G., Rao, V. M., Dalinka, M., et al. (1986): Hematopoietic and fatty bone marrow distribution in the normal and ischemic hip: New observations with 1.5-T MR imaging. *Radiology*, 161:199–202.
12. Mitchell, D. G., Rao, V., Dalinka, M., et al. (1986): MRI of joint fluid in the normal and ischemic hip. *AJR*, 146:1215–1218.
13. Per-Lennart, W., Bronstein, S. L., and Liedberg, J. (1986): Temporomandibular joint: Correlation between single-contrast videoarthrography and postmortem morphology. *Radiology*, 160:767–771.

14. Rao, V. M., Dalinka, M. K., Mitchell, D. G., et al. (1986): Osteopetrosis: MR characteristics at 1.5 T. *Radiology,* 161:217–220.
15. Rao, V. M., Fishman, M., Mitchell, D. G., et al. (1986): Painful sickle cell crisis: Bone marrow patterns observed with MR imaging. *Radiology,* 161:211–215.
16. Reicher, M., et al. (1986): Meniscal injuries: Detection using MR imaging. *Radiology,* 159:753–758.
17. Richardson, M. L., Amparo, E. G., Helms, C. A., et al. (1985): Theoretical considerations for optimizing contrast between primary musculoskeletal tumors and normal tissue with spin-echo magnetic resonance imaging. *Invest. Radiol.,* 20:492.
18. Richardson, M. L., Kilcoyne, R. F., Gillespy, T., et al. (1986): Magnetic resonance imaging of musculoskeletal neoplasms. *Radiol. Clin. North Am.,* 24:259–267.

Artifacts

1. Babcock, E. E., Brateman, L., Weinreb, J. C., et al. (1985): Edge artifacts in MR images. *JCAT,* 9:252–257.
2. Bradley, W. G., Waluch, V., Lai, K. S., et al. (1984): The appearance of rapidly flowing blood on magnetic resonance images. *AJR,* 143:1167–1174.
3. Feinberg, D. A., Hoenninger, J. C., Crooks, L. E., et al. (1985): Inner volume MR imaging: Technical concepts and their application. *Radiology,* 156:743–747.
4. Lukeke, K. M., Roschmann, P., and Tischler, R. (1985): Susceptibility artifacts in NMR imaging. *Magn. Reson. Imag.* 3(4):329–343.
5. Maudsley, A. A., Simon, H. E., and Hilal, S. K. (1984): Magnetic field measurement by NMR imaging. *J. Phys. E: Sci. Instrum.,* 17:216–220.
6. Moran, P. R., Moran, R. A., and Karstaedt, N. (1985): Verification and evaluation of internal flow and motion. True magnetic resonance imaging by the phase gradient modulation method. *Radiology,* 154:433–441.
7. O'Donnell, M., and Edelstein, W. A. (1985): NMR imaging in the presence of magnetic field inhomogeneities and gradient field nonlinearities. *Med. Phys.,* 12:20–26.
8. Porter, B. A., Hastrup, W., Richardson, M. L., et al. (1987): Classification and investigation of artifacts in magnetic resonance imaging. *RadioGraphics,* 7(2):271–287.
9. Pusey, E., Lufkin, R. B., Brown, R. K. J., et al. (1986): Magnetic resonance imaging artifacts: Mechanism and clinical significance. *RadioGraphics,* 6(5):891–911.
10. Schultz, C. L., Alfidi, R. J., Nelson, A. D., et al. (1984): The effect of motion on two-dimensional Fourier transformation magnetic resonance images. *Radiology,* 152:117–121.
11. Soila, K. P., Viamonte, J., Jr., and Starewiez, P. M. (1984): Chemical shift mis-registration effect in magnetic resonance imaging. *Radiology,* 153:819–820.
12. Sze, G., DeArmond, S. J., Brant-Zawadzki, M., et al. (1986): Foci of MRI signal (pseudo lesions) anterior to the frontal horns: Histologic correlations of a normal finding. *AJR,* 147:331–337.
13. Weinreb, J. C., Brateman, L., Babcock, E. E., et al. (1985): Chemical shift artifact in clinical magnetic resonance images at 0.35T. *AJR,* 145:183–185.
14. Wood, M. L., and Henkelman, R. M. (1985): MR image artifacts from periodic motion. *Med. Phys.,* 12:143–151.
15. Wood, M. L., and Henkelman, R. M. (1985): Truncation artifacts in MR imaging. *Magn. Reson. Med.,* 2:517–526.

CHAPTER 7

1. Bradley, W. G., Jr. (1986): Comparing costs and efficacy of MRI. *AJR,* 146:1307–1310.
2. Bradley, W. G., Jr., Waluch, V., Yadley, R. A., and Wycoff, R. R. (1984): Comparison of CT and MR in 400 patients with suspected disease of the brain and cervical spinal cord. *Radiology,* 152:695–702.
3. Citrin, C. M. (1987): Around-the-clock operation keeps throughput high at MR center. *Diagnostic Imaging,* 166.

4. De Wolfe, A. (1987): Good marketing a key ingredient to a successful imaging center. *Diagnostic Imaging*, 137–142.
5. Doubilet, P. M. (1987): "Cost Effective": A trendy, often misused term. *AJR*, 148:827–828.
6. Drew, P. G. (1986): MRI equipment prices will fall as competition heats up. *Diagnostic Imaging*, 192–193.
7. Droege, R. T., Ekstrand, K. E., and Coffey, C. W., II (1986): Systems components for consideration in purchasing an NMR imager. *RadioGraphics*, 6(1):154–159.
8. Evens, R. G. (1987): An efficacy lesson for medical radiologists from our dental colleagues. *Radiology*, 162:873.
9. Evens, R. G. (1984): Computed tomography—a controversy revisited. *N. Engl. J. Med.*, 310:1183–1185.
10. Evens, R. G. (1986): The diffusion of MRI in the United States: What is fact and what is speculation. *AJR*, 147:856–857.
11. Fullerton, G. D. (1987): Users of MRI finally entering phase of realistic optimism. *Diagnostic Imaging*, 87.
12. Graham, J. (1986): Wall Street analyst predicts 16% of nation's beds will shut by 1990. *Modern Healthcare*, 90–92.
13. Hasegawa, J., Iriguchi, N., Ueshima, Y., et al. (1987): Natural abundance carbon-13 NMR imaging of the human arm. Presented at SMRM meeting, San Antonio.
14. Hayes, R. H. (1985): Strategic planning—forward in reverse? *Harvard Business Review*, 111–119.
15. Hess, T. P. (1987): In southern California, MRI attracts more patients than centers can handle. *Diagnostic Imaging*, 53–61.
16. Hopkins, A. L., Barr, R. G., and Bratton, C. B. (1987): Contrast agents based on oxygen-17. Presented at SMRM meeting, San Antonio.
17. James, A. E., Carroll, F., Pickens, D. R., et al. (1986): Medical image management. *Radiology*, 160:847–851.
18. James, A. E., Jr., Partain, C. L., Patton, J. A., et al. (1985): Marshall Eskridge Lecture: Current status of magnetic resonance imaging. *South. Med. J.*, 78:580–597.
19. Johnson, K. C., and Bradley, W. G. (1986): Identify true costs of services in drawing up MRI business plan. *Diagnostic Imaging*, 73–81.
20. Levy, J. M., and Hessel, S. J. (1987): Equipment purchasing a top concern among community-based radiologists. *Diagnostic Imaging*, 91–93.
21. Macapinlac, H., Engelstad, B., Ramos, E., et al. (1987): Fe-HBED and Fe-EHPG: Iron complexes exhibiting hepatobiliary enhancement in MRI. Presented at SMRM meeting, San Antonio.
22. Muroff, L. R. (1987): The economic outlook for radiologists and diagnostic imaging. Presented at Economics of Diagnostic Imaging 1987: National symposium, New Orleans.
23. Muroff, L. (1987): Socioeconomic issues. Presented at SMRM meeting, San Antonio.
24. Nishimura, D. G., Pauly, J. M., Macovski, A., et al. (1987): Magnetic resonance angiography. Presented at SMRM meeting, San Antonio.
25. Office of Technology Assessment (1984): Medical technology and costs of the Medicare program. Publication no. OTA-H-227. U.S. Government Printing Office, Washington, D.C.
26. Peddecord, K. M., Janon, E. A., and Robins, J. M. (1987): Use of MR imaging in an outpatient MR center. *AJR*, 148:809–812.
27. Petitti, D. B. (1986): Competing technologies: Implications for the costs and complexity of medical care. *N. Engl. J. Med.*, 315(23):1480–1483.
28. Ratner, A. V., Parish, D., Bradley-Simpson, B., et al. (1987): Rapidly sequential flourine and proton magnetic resonance imaging using a variable magnetic field strength approach. Presented at SMRM meeting, San Antonio.
29. Ratner, A. V., Sotak, C., Muller, H., et al. (1987): ^{19}F in vivo spectroscopy of neoplasms. Presented at SMRM meeting, San Antonio.
30. Schroeder, S. A. (1985): Magnetic resonance imaging: present costs and potential gains. *Ann. Intern. Med.*, 102:551–553.
31. Sisk, J. E. (1984): Effects of increased competition in health care on the use and innovation of medical technology. *Health Care Manage. Rev.*, 9(3):21–34.
32. Sotak, C. H., Chew, W. M., Mills, P. A., et al. (1987): In vivo ^{19}F NMR study of halothane elimination from the rabbit brain using the isis spatial localization technique. Presented at SMRM meeting, San Antonio.

33. Steinberg, E. P., Sisk, J. E., and Locke, K. E. (1985): X-ray CT and magnetic resonance imagers: Diffusion patterns and policy issues. *N. Eng. J. Med.*, 313(14):859–864.
34. Young, S. W. (1987): Practicing MRI in the changing economic environment. Presented at SMRM meeting, San Antonio.
35. Young, S. W., and Bartrum, R. J., Jr. (1984): *Financial Independence—A Doctor's Guide.* Raven Press, New York.

CHAPTER 8

1. Bottomley, P. A., Rogers, H. H., and Foster, T. H. (1986): NMR imaging shows water distribution and transport in plant root systems in situ. *Proc. Natl. Acad. Sci. USA*, 83:87–89.
2. Bottomley, P. A., Edelstein, W. A., Foster, T. H., and Adams, W. A. (1985): In vivo solvent-suppressed localized hydrogen NMR spectroscopy: A window to metabolism? *Proc. Natl. Acad. Sci. USA*, 82:2148–2151.
3. Bottomley, P. A., et al. (1985): Noninvasive detection and monitoring of regional myocardial ischemia in situ using depth-resolved ^{31}P NMR spectroscopy. *Proc. Natl. Acad. Sci. USA*, 82:8747–8751.
4. Bottomley, P. A., Foster, T. H., and Leue, W. M. (1984): In vivo nuclear magnetic resonance chemical shift imaging by selective irradiation. *Proc. Natl. Acad. Sci. USA*, 81:6856–6860.
5. Bottomley, P. A., Hardy, C. J., Argersinger, R. E., and Allen-More, G. (1987): A review of ^{1}H nuclear magnetic resonance relaxation in pathology: Are T_1 and T_2 diagnostic? *Med. Phys.* 14(1):1–37.
6. Bottomley, P. A., Smith, L. S., Leue, W. M., and Charles, C. (1985): Slice-interleaved depth-resolved surface-coil spectroscopy (SLIT DRESS) for rapid ^{31}P NMR in vivo. *J. Magn. Reson.*, 64:347–351.
7. DeLaPaz, R. L., Bernstein, R., Dave, J. V., and Chang, P. J. (1986): Tissue characterization with MRI using advanced digital processing techniques ("fuzzy" clustering). In: *Abstracts of the Society of Magnetic Resonance in Medicine, 5th Annual Meeting, Montreal.*
8. Wolf, W., Albright, M. J., Silver, M. S., et al. (1987): Fluorine-19 NMR spectroscopic studies of the metabolism of 5-fluorouracil in the liver of patients undergoing chemotherapy. *Magn. Reson. Imag.*, 5(3):1–5.

CHAPTER 9

1. American National Standards Institute (1982): Safety levels with respect to human exposure to radiofrequency fields, 300 kHz to 100 GHz. Report no. ANSI C95.1-1982, Institute of Electrical and Electronic Engineers, New York.
2. Bottomley, P. A., and Andrew, E. R. (1978): RF magnetic field penetration, phase shift, and power dissipation in biological tissue: implications for NMR imaging. *Phys. Med. Biol.*, 23:630–643.
3. Bottomley, P. A., and Edelstein, W. A. (1981): Power deposition in whole-body NMR imaging. *Med. Phys.*, 8:510–512.
4. Bottomley, P. A., Redington, R. W., Edelstein, W. A., and Schenck, J. F. (1985): Estimating radiofrequency power deposition in body NMR imaging. *Magn. Reson. Med.*, 2:336–349.
5. Brody, A. S., Sorette, M. P., Gooding, C. A., et al. (1985): Induced alignment of flowing sickle erythrocytes in a magnetic field. *Invest. Radiol.*, 20:560–566.
6. Budinger, T. F. (1981): Nuclear magnetic resonance in vivo studies: Known thresholds for health effects. *JCAT*, 5:800–811.
7. Fowler, J. R., ter Penning, B., Syverud, S. A., and Levy, R. C. (1986): Magnetic field hazard. *N. Engl. J. Med.*, 34(23):1517.
8. Shellock, F. G., and Crues, J. V. (1987): Temperature, heart rate, and blood pressure changes associated with clinical MR imaging at 1.5 T. *Radiology,* 163:259–262.
9. Spiegel, R. F., Deffbaugh, D. M., and Mann, J. E. (1980): A thermal model of the human body exposed to an electromagnetic field. *Bioelectromagnetics,* 1:253–270.

Appendix I

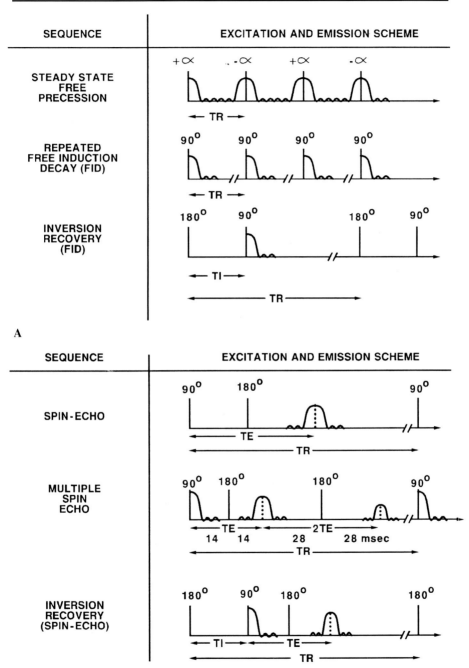

FIG. I.1. Schematic representation of RF excitation-and-emission sequence.

Appendix II

American College of Radiology Imaging Definitions

Partial saturation

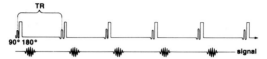

Sequence illustrated with 0.2 S TR (approximately 7 msec elapses between the 90° and 180° pulses)

Inversion recovery

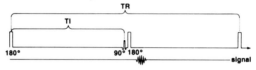

Sequence illustrated with 1.0 S TR and 500 msec TI

Spin echo

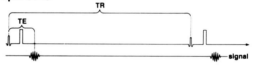

Sequence illustrated with 0.8 S TR and 100 msec TE (approximately 50 ms elapses between the 90° and 180° pulses)

Multiple echo

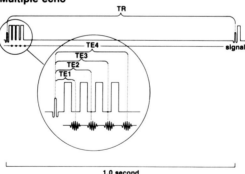

Sequence illustrated with 1.0 S TR and TE of 25, 50, 75 and 100 msec.

FIG. II.1. Repetition time (TR): the period of time between the beginning of a pulse sequence and the beginning of a succeeding (essentially identical) pulse sequence. Inversion time (T_1): the time between the middle of an inverting RF pulse and the middle of a subsequent 90° pulse to detect the amount of longitudinal magnetization. Echo time (TE): the time between the middle of a 90° pulse and the middle of spin-echo production. For multiple echoes, use TE_1, TE_2, etc. (Courtesy of the General Electric Co.)

Atlas of Normal MRI Anatomy

This atlas shows a series of illustrations of normal anatomy. They should be used in conjunction with the figures in the preceding chapters in order to follow the normal anatomy through a series of contiguous slices. Generalized sequences are included to provide an overall view of gross anatomic relationships. Some detailed views of specific anatomic areas are included to further define important clinical anatomic relationships. Normal anatomy is illustrated throughout the book, however, this should provide the reader with supplemental images useful in interpreting the images presented in the text.

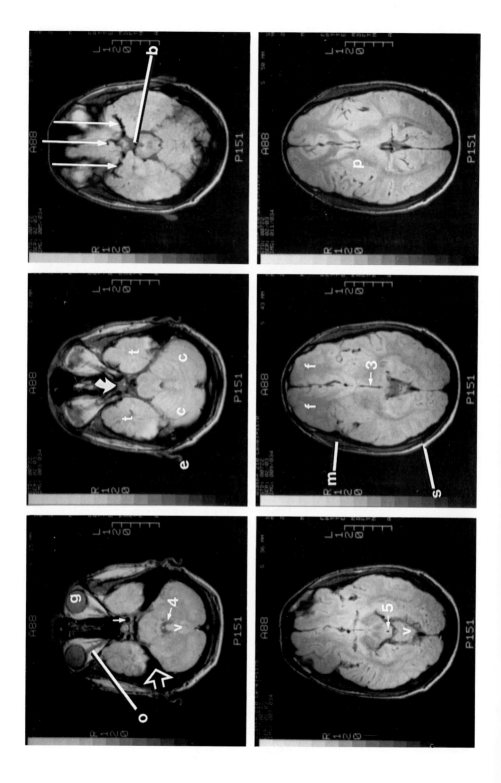

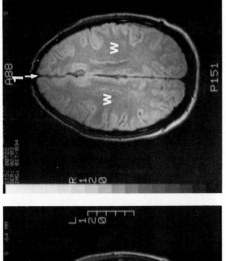
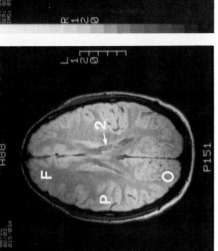
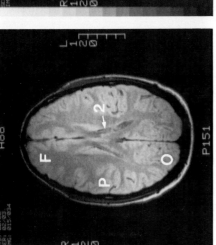

FIG. A.1. A series of 5-mm axial images from the top of the lateral ventricles to the level of the optic globes: (g) optic globe; (o) optic nerve; (v) vermis of the cerebellum; *(open arrow)* external auditory canal (the arrow is placed over the bone of the mastoid air cells on the right); *(small arrow)* left internal carotid artery (note the pituitary gland between the two carotid arteries); (t) temporal lobe; (c) cerebellum; (e) pinna of the ear; *(curved arrow)* pituitary gland (note the ophthalmic arteries taking origin from the internal carotid on either side of the curved white arrow); *(long white arrows)* anterior portion of the circle of Willis including the left and right middle cerebral and the two anterior cerebral arteries; (b) basilar artery (just anterior to the pons; note the aqueduct within the pons just anterior to the vermis and the *small black circle* and the paired low-intensity structures representing the red nucleus and the substantia nigra within the pons; (m) bone marrow within the skull; (s) subcutaneous fat; (f) frontal lobes; (p) putamen [note the anterior and posterior limbs of the internal capsule (V-shaped low-intensity structure) surrounding the putamen]; (x) corpus callosum, anterior commissure; (z) corpus callosum, splenium; (n) caudate nucleus; (T) thalamus; (F) frontal lobe; (P) parietal lobe; (O) occipital lobe; (w) white matter (corona radiata) in this balanced image is seen as a lower-intensity structure, with surrounding cortical gray matter seen as a structure of slightly higher intensity; the low intensity seen between the convolutions of the gray matter represents CSF contained in the cerebral convolutions; (1) interhemispheric fissure; (2) left lateral ventricle; (3) third ventricle; (4) fourth ventricle; (5) aqueduct of Sylvius (1.5 T, 2000/25).

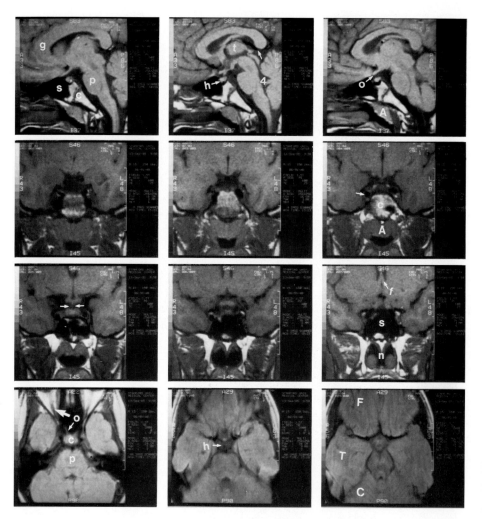

FIG. A.2. Sagittal (**top row**), coronal (**middle two rows**), and axial (**bottom row**) detailed views through the pituitary gland. These sections were obtained from a 15-year-old male using a partial-saturation sequence: (g) genu of the corpus callosum (note splenium of the corpus callosum posteriorly), which is just above the internal cerebral veins and great cerebral vein; (p) pons; (c) clivus; (s) sphenoid sinus (note the left optic nerve at the superior portion of the sphenoid sinus in the first image); (t) thalamus; (h) pituitary gland; (4) fourth ventricle (note the cerebellum posteriorly and the pons anteriorly; the prepontine cistern anterior to the pons has dark structures within it that represent flow voids from the serpiginous basilar artery); (*arrow,* middle top row) internal cerebral veins joining to form the great cerebral vein just inferior and posterior to the splenium of the corpus callosum; the septum pellucidum is seen just above the thalamus; (o) optic nerve; (A) adenoids in the posterior nasal pharynx; (*arrow,* coronal image) right internal carotid artery (the left internal carotid artery is a low-intensity circular structure on the other side of the clivus); (*paired arrows*) the hypophyseal stalk, with the pituitary gland below (between both carotid arteries and above the sphenoid sinus). Note the optic chiasm above the internal carotid arteries passing through the cavernous sinus and, although they are not shown well, the third cranial nerve above the carotids and the sixth cranial nerve and first and second divisions of the fifth cranial nerve inferior to the carotid arteries on either side of the sphenoid sinus.

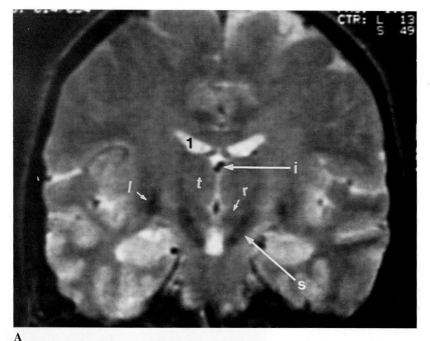

A

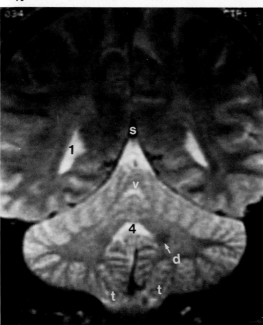

B

FIG. A.3. Coronal T$_2$-weighted MR images (2,000/80) through the third ventricle (A) and through the fourth ventricle and the cerebellum (B) illustrating some of the cerebral nuclei: (1) lateral ventricles; (4) fourth ventricle; (i) internal cerebral veins; (t) thalamus; (r) red nucleus; (s) substantia nigra; (l) lenticulate nucleus; (d) dentate nucleus; (v) vermis; (s) straight sinus; (t) cerebellar tonsil.

FIG. A.2. (continued) The third ventricle and lateral ventricles are seen as low-intensity structures above the optic chiasm; (f) fornix (note the lateral ventricles above and a portion of the third ventricle below); (n) the nasal passage, with the inferior concha on either side of the n; (F) frontal lobe in the anterior cranial fossa; (T) temporal lobe in the middle cranial fossa; (C) cerebellum in the posterior cranial fossa. Note the well-defined circle of Willis in the last axial cut, bottom row, with the posterior cerebral arteries passing posteriorly around the pons.

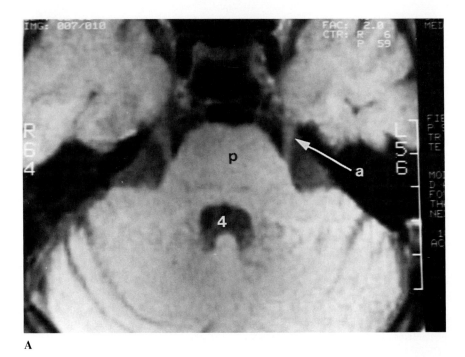

A

FIG. A.4. Cranial nerves of the pons, lower pons, and medulla oblongata shown on axial views of the pons (**A** & **B**) and the medulla oblongata (**C**), demonstrating the sixth through ninth cranial nerves; (a) abducens nerve (VI); (f) facial (VII); (c, *large arrow*) vestibulocochlear nerve (VIII); (*arrowhead*) a rootlet of the glossopharyngeal nerve (IX); (p) pons; (4) fourth ventricle; (c, *small arrow*) cochlea; (v) vestibular apparatus; (m) medulla oblongata; (O) olive; (P) pyramid.

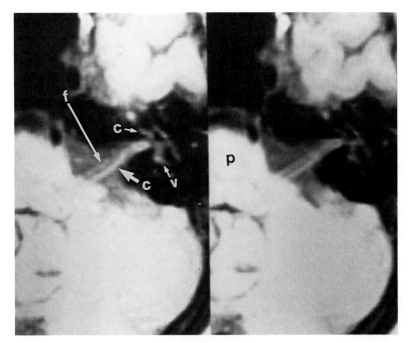

B

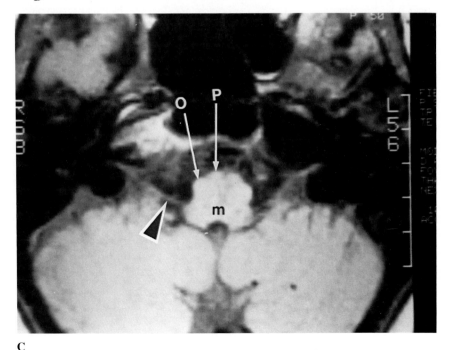

C

FIG. A.4. continued.

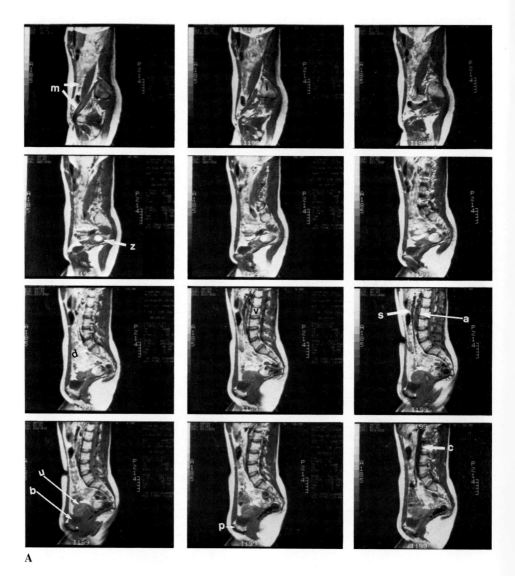

A

FIG. A.5. Sagittal (**A**), coronal (**B**), and axial (**C**) series of sequential 5-mm MR images (1,600/25) from a normal 20-year-old woman: (m) psoas and iliacus muscle; (i) iliac bone; (z) high-intensity material contained in the sigmoid colon; (d) intervertebral disc spaces; (v) marrow within the vertebral body; (a) aorta; (s) superior mesenteric artery; (c) inferior vena cava; (u) uterus; (b) bladder; (p) pubic symphyses; (k) left kidney.

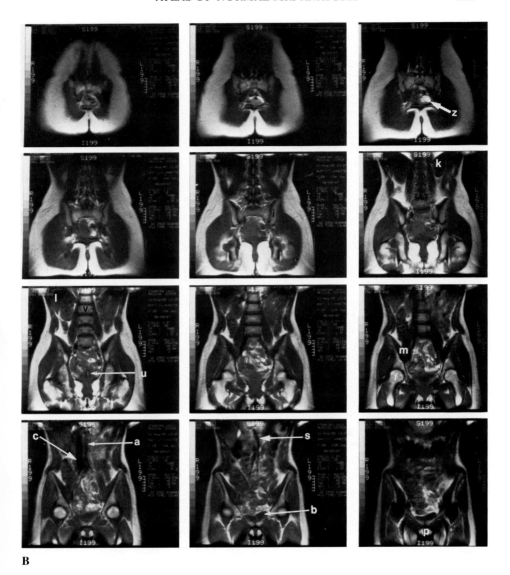

B

FIG. A.5. continued.

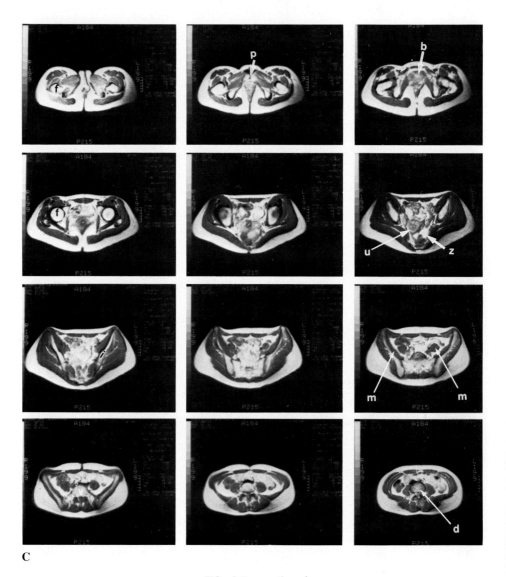

C

FIG. A.5. continued.

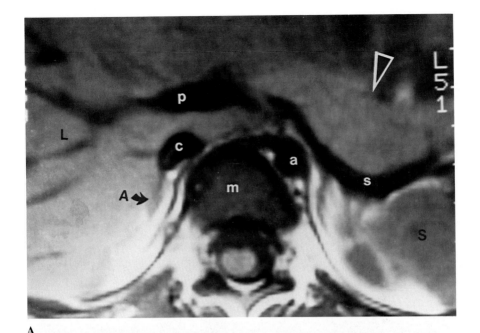

A

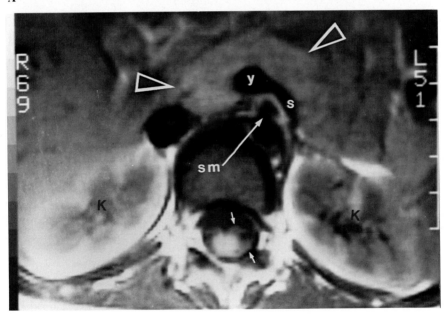

B

FIG. A.6. Partial-saturation detailed studies of the anatomy in the vicinity of the pancreas. Signal-intensity falloff from posterior to anterior is due to the surface coil used in this study; (p) portal vein; (c) inferior vena cava; (a) aorta; (s) splenic vein; (y) confluence of the splenic vein and portal vein; (sm) the origin of the superior mesenteric artery from the aorta; (m) bone marrow within the vertebral body; the low-intensity signal circumferentially around this is due to the cortical bone of the vertebral body. Note curvilinear tubular structures representing the paravertebral venous plexus: (L) liver; (A) right adrenal; (S) spleen (inferior pole); (k) kidneys; (*arrowheads*) pancreas; (*small arrows*) dorsal and ventral nerve roots from the spinal cord.

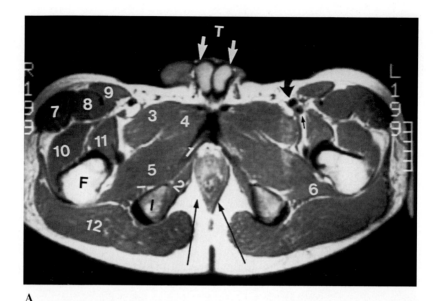

A

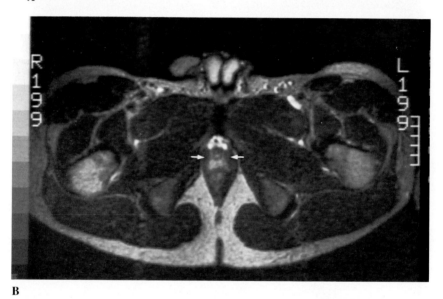

B

FIG. A.7. First- and second-echo axial images from a normal male pelvis (**A & B**, 1,600/40/70). Note the normal prostate, with high-intensity central paraurethral zone, a lower-intensity central zone, and a higher-intensity peripheral zone that is best seen on the second echo (**B**, *arrows*). Also note the chemical-shift artifact around the levator ani muscle (*long black arrows*) caused by the juxtaposition of water-containing muscle and surrounding pararectal fat. The normal testicles (T) are seen anteriorly, and the femoral artery (*curved black arrow*) and vein (*short black arrow*) and ischial tuberosity (I) are marked; (1) external oblique; (2) internal oblique; (3) pectineus; (4) adductor brevis; (5) adductor minimus; (6) quadratus femoris; (7) tensor fascia lata; (8) rectus femoris; (9) sartorius; (10) vastus lateralis; (11) iliopsoas; (12) gluteus maximus. Note also the phase-encoded artifact emanating from the femoral arteries and veins on the second echo (**B**) seen as vertical lines of noise through the respective vessels.

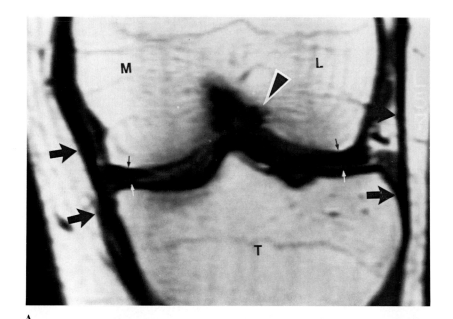

A

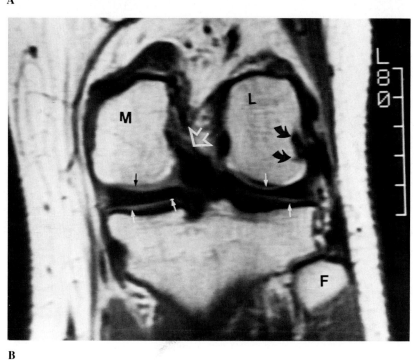

B

FIG. A.8. Coronal (**A** & **B**) and sagittal (**C–F**) images from a normal knee.

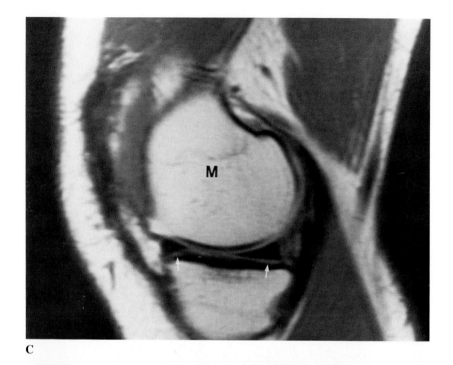

C

D

FIG. A.8. continued.

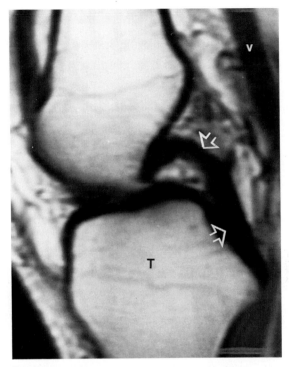

E

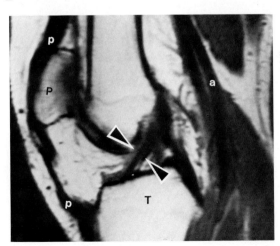

F

FIG. A.8. *(continued)* The coronal views were obtained through the anterior (**A**) and posterior (**B**) knee joint, and the sagittal views were obtained to demonstrate the medial and lateral menisci (**C** & **D**) and the posterior and anterior cruciate ligaments (**E** & **F**). The lateral femoral condyle describes a logarithmic spiral in its perimeter configuration, and this can be of help in evaluating sagittal views of the knee when the fibula is not in view (**F**) or when only the medial condyle is shown.

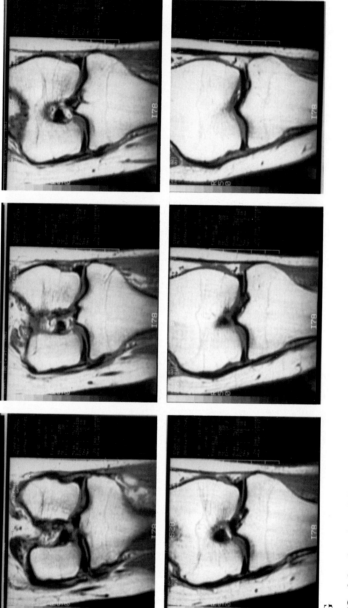

FIG. A.8. *(continued)* Coronal (**G**) and sagittal (**H**) contiguous sections through a normal knee are for comparison with (**A–F**). The images progress from posterior to anterior (coronal) and lateral to medial (sagittal) (1,500/20). (**L**) lateral femoral condyle; (**M**) medial femoral condyle; (**T**) tibia; (**F**) fibula; (**P**) patella; (**p**) patellar tendon; (**v**) popliteal vein. The menisci (*short arrows*), the posterior cruciate ligament (*open arrows*), the anterior cruciate ligament (*arrowheads*), the medial and lateral collateral ligaments (*black arrowheads*), and the tendinous insertion of the lateral head of the gastrocnemius muscle (*curved black arrows*) are also indicated.

G

270

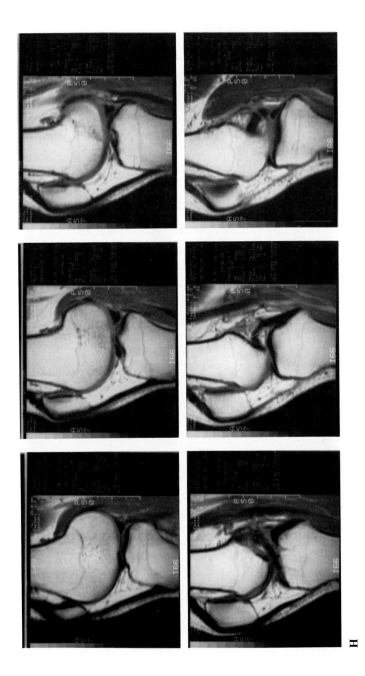

H

271

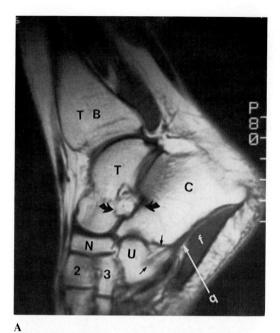

A

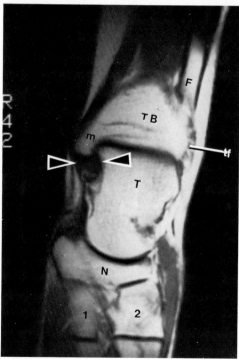

B

FIG. A.9. Sagittal (**A**) and coronal (**B**) partial-saturation images through the mid-plane of the normal ankle; (TB) tibia; (T) thallus; (C) calcaneus; (F) fibula; (N) navicular; (U) cuboid; (f) flexor digitorum brevis muscle; (q) quadratus plantae muscle; (m) medial malleolus; (tf) inferior tibiofibular ligament; (*curved black arrows*) tarsal sinus (tunnel) containing the interosseous talocalcaneal ligament and fat; (*small black arrows*) plantar calcaneocuboid ligament (short plantar ligament); (*arrowheads*) deltoid ligament; (1, 2, and 3) first, second, and third cuneiform bones that articulate with the first, second, and third metatarsals.

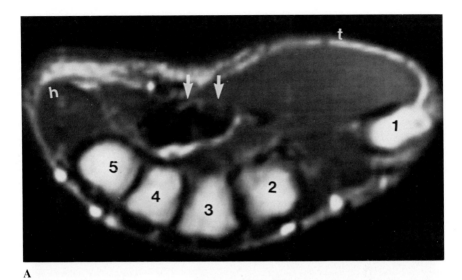

A

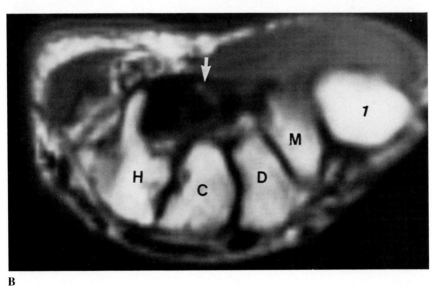

B

FIG. A.10. Axial MR images through a normal right hand, beginning distally in the meta-carpals (**A**) and progressing superiorly to the radial ulnar joint (**D**). The hand is mounted with the volar surface up; (1–5) first (thumb) through fifth (little finger) carpal bones; (M) trape-zium; (D) trapezoid; (C) capitate; (H) hamate; (S) scaphoid; (L) lunate; (Q) triquetrum; (P) pisiform; (R) radius; (U) ulna; (t) thenar eminence; (h) hypothenar eminence; (*arrows*) flexor tendons of the hand in the flexor retinaculum passing through the carpal tunnel.

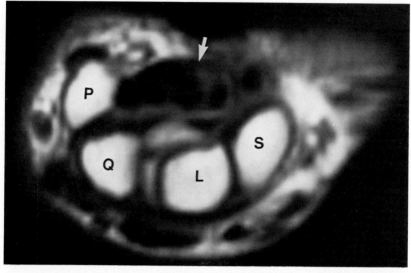

C

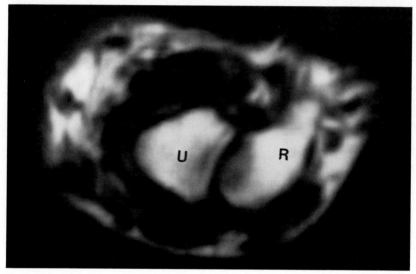

D

FIG. A.10.   continued.

Subject Index

A

Abdomen, 5
  artifact, 149
  vascular patency, 157
Abdominal mass, 164
Absorption line, 239
Adenoma
  pituitary, 104
  recurrent, 107–108
Adiabatic fast passage, 239
Adnexal cyst, 165–166
Adrenal gland, 157, 161
Agricultural applications, 202–204
AIDS, 109, 110
Aliasing, 177–184
Alzheimer's disease, 100
American College of Radiology Imaging, 254
Amyloid angiopathy, 113
Anatomy, normal, 129, 255–274
Aneursym, great vein of Galen, 140
Aneurysm, ferromagnetic clip, 101–113
Angiomyolipoma, 79, 154
Angiopathy
  amyloid, 113
  congophillic, 113
Angular frequency, 35, 239
Angular magnetic moment, 28
Angular momentum, 28
Anisotropy, 236
Ankle, 272
Anterior cruciate ligament, ruptured, 180
Aortic arch, 132
Aortic dissection, 126, 132
  artifact, 182
Architectural requirements, 230–231
Arteriovenous malformation, 12
Artery, 2, 4
Articular eminens, 6–7
Artifact, 177–188
  abdomen, 149
  aortic dissection, 182
  bounce-point, 188

brainstem, 177–184
carcinoma, 185
cardiovascular, 149
cerebellum, 177–184, 188
cervical spine, 183
chemical-shift, 184–185
flow-related, 115
inhomogeneity, 11
  magnetic, 177
metallic, 184, 185
motion, 177
over-range, 1
pelvis, 149
pulsation-motion, 183
radial, 189
radio-frequency field, 185–186
respiratory, 149
sources, 177
static-electric-discharge, 188
subglottic stenosis, 183
wraparound, 177–184
zero-line, 186
Aseptic necrosis, 172, 176
Astrocytoma, 104
  recurrent, 218–219
Auditory canal, 5
  external, 6–7
  internal, 5
Axillary vein occlusion, 145
Axis, phase-encoded, 73–75

B

Back-projection reconstruction, 69, 70
  filtered, 70–71
  multiple-angle, 69
Baker's cyst, 179
Basilar vein, 11
Bilaminar zone, 6–7
Biological research, 193
Bladder, 262–264
Blood, 138–149
  clotted, 148–149

Paramagnetic resonance, electron, 29
Paramagnetic species, 82–84
Parkinson's disease, 100, 161
Partial saturation, 254
Partial saturation method, 64
Particle, spinning, 28–29
Particulate contrast agent, 99–100
Patella, 150
Patient demographics, 192, 193
Pelvic mass, 165–166
Pelvis, 5
  artifact, 149
  male, 266
Perfluorooctyl bromide, 208
Petroleum tertiary-recovery study, 203
Phase coherence, 47
Phase encoding, 72–75
Phase-angle encoding, 146
Phase-display approach of Wideen, 147
Phase-encoded axis, 73–75
Phase-encoding imaging, 69
Phosphorus, 1
Physician, 192, 193
Physician income, 191
Pituitary, 112
Pituitary adenoma, 104
Pituitary gland, 258
Polar coordinate, 40
Pons, 260–261
Position-emission tomography, 217
Postoperative patient, 115
Power source, alternating current, 19–20
Precession, 32–36, 241
Precessional frequency, 34–36
Probe, 241
Professional fee, 191
Prostatic carcinoma, 168, 185
Proton, 28–29, 31, 54–55
  antiparallel, 32–35
    precession, 35–36
  coherent, 142
  magnetic dipole, 32
  magnetic resonance, 54–55
  parallel, 32–35
    precession, 35–36
Proton density, 41
Proton imaging, high-resolution, 217, 219
Psoas muscle, 162–163, 262–264
Pubic symphysis, 262–264
Pulmonary artery, 93, 131, 133
Pulsation-motion artifact, 183
Pulse sequence, 64, 241
  gray scale, 80

Q
Quadriceps femorus, 14–15
Quadriceps tendon, 180
Quenching, 241

R
Radial artifact, 189
Radiation, 1
Radio frequency, 241
Radio wave, 24–26
Radio-frequency coil, 19–20, 242. *See also*
    Specific type
  schematic, 19
Radio-frequency field artifact, 185–186
Radio-frequency magnetic field, 229
  artificial pacemaker, 229
  heating, 229
  safety, 229–230
Radio-frequency pulse, 242
Radio-frequency signal, 37
Readout gradient, frequency-encoded, 73–77
Reduced-flip-angle/gradient-reversal
    technique, 143
Referral, 194
Relaxation, 242
Relaxation time, 1, 23, 41, 42
  contrast agent, 100
  determinants, 83–98
Renal image, 206–207
Renal vein, 13
Renal vein thrombosis, 157–160
Repetition rate, 64
Repetition time, 242
  gray scale, 80–81
Research funding, 193
Resistance, 19–20
Resonance, 24, 29–30, 242
Resonant frequency, 34–36
Respiratory motion, thorax, 115–126
Reticuloendothelial system, 99–100
Retina, ferromagnetic clip, 101–113
Review quiz, 237–238
Rhabdomyosarcoma, 134–135
Rotating frame, 242
Rotational correlation time, 96–97

S
Saddle-shaped coil, 19–20
Safety, 227–236
Sarcoidosis, 112